ONE MOMENT CHANGES EVERYTHING

The All-America Tragedy of Don Rogers

SEAN D. HARVEY

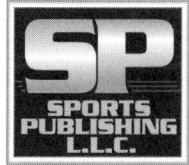

SportsPublishingLLC.com

ISBN-13: 978-1-59670-231-8

© 2007 by Sean D. Harvey

All rights reserved. Except for use in a review, no part of this publication may be reproduced, stored in or introduced into a retrieval system, or transmitted, in any form or by any means (electronic, mechanical, xerography, photocopy, recording or otherwise), without prior written permission of both the copyright owner and the publisher of this book. The scanning, uploading, and distribution of this book via the Internet or via any other means without the permission of the publisher is illegal and punishable by law.

Publishers: Peter L. Bannon and Joseph J. Bannon Sr.
Senior managing editor: Susan M. Moyer
Editor: Travis W. Moran
Art director: Dustin J. Hubbart
Cover design: Dustin J. Hubbart
Project manager: Kathryn R. Holleman
Photo editor: Erin Linden-Levy

Sports Publishing L.L.C.
804 North Neil Street
Champaign, IL 61820
Phone: 1-877-424-2665
Fax: 217-363-2073
www.SportsPublishingLLC.com

Printed in the United States of America

CIP data available upon request.

To my father and mother: a writer and an artist.

PREFACE

On the various lists of the most profound and painful sports tragedies of all time, the June 27, 1986, death of Don Rogers ranks near the top or is somehow excluded all together. His schizophrenic standing is complicated and varied, but primarily has to do with the combination of the *cause* of Rogers' death—a drug overdose—and the *timing* of his passing—just one week after University of Maryland basketball superstar Len Bias perished, seemingly from the same cause. The later rise and fall of Don's younger brother, Reggie, a 1987 first-round NFL draft pick of the Detroit Lions, have, in the minds of some, further disqualified this enigmatic family—specifically, Don Rogers—from any list that is intended to evoke fond memory.

Yet, one fact remains consistent to all those who view Don with unsympathetic eyes, and that is: Most who have formed that rigid opinion do not know the entire story of Don Rogers, the great UCLA and Cleveland Browns' safety, the much loved family man. In places like Cleveland, as well as up and down the West Coast, Don's legacy as a community leader and a football star are secure. Just over 20 years since his death, many people still are overcome by emotion and sadness at the mere mention of his name.

However, admittedly, it is complicated. Don died doing something out of character, and, undeniably, he died doing something needless and naive: cocaine. What followed was a firestorm of events that wracked his supremely talented family, affected massive changes to the very laws of America, and transformed the NCAA and its relationship to student athletes as well as to sports agents altogether—

not to mention those who introduced as antagonists here, who were supported by the Mafia. Lastly, Don's death doomed a rising NFL franchise to a series of heartbreaking near misses as they thrice fell just one victory shy of the Super Bowl.

The message of Don's story is clear: One moment changes everything. Good luck and bad luck, momentum and inertia, every fork in the road—everything hangs on individual instances of choice. The right decision leads to promise, and the wrong decision could catalyze catastrophe. Don Rogers' death affects us all to this very day, whether we watch sports or not. It serves as a reminder—a reminder that blood, community, and above all, humanity link us all. It is a reminder that if we hold perfect strangers to our highest standards and expect the best from them, we should hold ourselves to those same standards and expect the best from ourselves.

The man sitting next to you on the bus; the clean-up hitter for the New York Yankees; the cashier at the grocery store; the all-league safety for the Cleveland Browns, you, me—we may think we have little in common, but we are all linked. What we do and what others do, affects us all in ways that become apparent over time, as again and again, one act, one decision, and one seemingly inconsequential moment in time is shown to change everything.

ACKNOWLEDGMENTS

Completing any endeavor that requires extensive research usually results from a collective effort, and this book is no exception.

Considering this, I am profoundly grateful to Corey Mullins, Tracy Battistessa, and Katja Raesch, for their patience, advice, and guidance throughout the writing process.

I would also like to thank Travis Moran and Noah Amstadter of Sports Publishing LLC, professionals who were invaluable in bringing this story to print.

To Chris Iglesias, Cyd, and Rick Chambers, and Chris Harvey, thank you for your unwavering moral support.

To the late, great literary agent, Al Lowman, and his business partner, BG Dilworth, thank you for your sizeable efforts in helping create the proposal.

Thank you also to the staff at the *Sacramento Bee*—specifically photo editor Mark Morris and Amy Eckert—John Elstadt, University of California at Davis Special Archivist; and Ms. Daryl Morrison, Head of Special Collections at UC-Davis.

Additionally, this book could not have been completed without the volunteers who make up the Grant Union High School Alumni Association. We should all aspire to love our jobs as much as they love theirs.

I want to acknowledge the excellent staff at the State Library in Sacramento as well—unsung perfectionists who make history available to us all.

Appreciative bows go out to author and professor, Dwight McBride; author Thomas Clark author and *Vanity Fair* columnist Michael Lutin; *Chicago Sun-Times* columnist Chris Deluca; photographer Brad Starks; and Don Rogers' former coaches: Marty Schottenheimer, Carl Youngstrom, and Dale Burney.

Lastly, I stand to applaud the longtime residents of Del Paso Heights, who have remained loyal to their neighborhood. They have seen their community evolve into a welcoming place where people want to live—a place that, more than ever, Don Rogers would be proud to call home.

1

Tucked into the corner of Del Paso Heights in North Sacramento is a place called Strawberry Manor—and to grow up there, is to grow up in hell.

The name itself, "Strawberry Manor" is misleading, like trying to plug a shotgun blast to the stomach with a single ball of cotton. In 1986 it was the poorest neighborhood in Sacramento, and one of the worst in California. Drug dealers with walkie-talkies stood on corners watching for cops as emaciated crack addicts stumble around in a daze. Sometimes those addicts lie down on the sidewalk in front of Fairbanks Elementary School. Sometimes they don't get up. Unescorted children hurdle their bodies without even looking down.

Most of the apartment buildings in Strawberry Manor look like a Motel 6—that is, if Motel 6 painted their buildings institutional shades of faded pink or lime, and neglected to replace doors that have been kicked in by debt-collecting strongmen.

Those who live farther away, in the surrounding suburbs and towns of Sacramento—places like Rocklin, Granite Bay, and Carmichael, neighborhoods adorned with yards manicured by brown-skinned men who don't speak English—they don't come to Del Paso Heights. They don't even *drive* through here. To the more affluent, the less addicted, even for those who've managed to extract themselves from the poverty and move on from places like Del Paso Heights, Richmond, South Central Los Angeles, National City, Hunter's Point, or East Oakland, the names of these places conjure a single emotion: FEAR.

ONE MOMENT CHANGES EVERYTHING

It's the night of June 26, 1986, one week after Maryland basketball superstar and Boston Celtics first-round draft pick, Len Bias, has died of a cocaine overdose. The country is still in shock.

In North Sacramento, 3,000 light-years away from the University of Maryland, a man is driving over Del Paso Heights on the elevated freeway. It's dark, and as he glances down at what is known to locals simply as "The Heights," he thinks back to the time his eldest son had a high school football game down there. And on that night, how his little junior helped the Longhorns escape back to the suburbs with a loss. Ever since that night, though, the only contact he's had with this neighborhood is when he reads about a shooting in the morning paper; or, like now, when he's on his way home from work, and he looks down into the darkness from above. It's an "otherworld" down there. And even though he's safely up high, he can't get out of this area fast enough. On this mid-summer night—it's always nighttime when he passes through—the yellowish streetlamps seem like pinpricks in the darkness amongst the grainy scenery. They offer him no thoughts of safe haven from the dangers he imagines lurk in each shadow.

He turns down the radio and listens to the engine. Foreign-born, it purrs reliably; and he exhales because he wouldn't want to break down now—not here. In fact, he thinks he remembers a story about someone whose car did quit somewhere around here. It overheated, and the driver had to pull to the side of the road. Or maybe, he thinks, it was a woman. In any event, he immediately recalls that something bad happened to the driver. Yet, this man's car is nearly brand new, under warranty, and, in fact, it will be under warranty until he gets something else to drive.

So once again, for the however-many-times the man has driven over this part of town, he looks off into the darkness, and he thinks to himself, "I'm so goddamned glad I don't have to live down there."

But lots of people do live down there. Or rather, they endure as much as live. Like subjects in an involuntary social experiment, they endure existences eloquently dissected in articles written by sociologists and college professors: the great prognosticators and observers of America's urban life. The people down there survive amidst the judgments and expectations of high achievers who have been born and raised and educated elsewhere: armchair quarterbacks studying worlds they'll never really know. Indeed, many people live down there, and in a thousand other places exactly like the Strawberry Manor neighborhood of Del Paso Heights in North Sacramento.

It could be any time in the last 40 years. But, by chance, the man in his reliable car gazes down from the elevated freeway on the evening of June 26, 1986. Without knowing it, he's looking at the home of NFL star Donald Rogers, who, at 24 years of age, already has the weight of the world upon his shoulders. That weight, and the invisible, insidious burdens that he'll never reveal will cause Don Rogers—recent winner of the AFC Rookie of the Year award, MVP of the Rose Bowl, consensus All-American, Cleveland Browns first-round draft pick, loved and respected by all—to do something stupid.

But everyone has burdens. Everyone in Del Paso Heights, and everyone in the wealthier worlds outside of Strawberry Manor, they all face challenges. So, just from where does this weighty burden heaped upon young Don Rogers come?

To be sure, his problems are a short lifetime in the making. They have to do with guiding his younger brother, Reggie, and their sister, Jackie, around fallen addicts lying prone in the street. They have to do with his mother's poor heart, and the father he's never known. They have to do with old friends and distant relatives who all want money. They have to do with it being the eve of his wedding day. They have to do with poverty, and what it means to make something of one's self, and then to discover that somehow, it's still not nearly good enough. And lastly, the burdens he carries have something to do with what it means to feel terrible inside, at a time in his life when Don realizes he should feel great.

"Don was everybody's father, including mine," said his mother, Loretha.

"He was my bodyguard," echoed his sister, Jackie.

ONE MOMENT CHANGES EVERYTHING

The story of Don, Reggie, and Jackie Rogers has to begin somewhere. There's Fairbanks Elementary School, where dealers wait by the gates like hungry bears standing in a shallow, salmon-filled river. There's Little League, where Don is the pitcher and Reggie the catcher on the same team. There's Loretha, their mother, who was born in the Deep South, and makes it to every one of her children's games.

But the story really begins at Norte Del Rio High School, a place that, much like the surrounding neighborhood, had never really found anything in which to invest its pride. Norte Del Rio High was comprised of mostly inexpensive, portable buildings, and had playing fields that were as much dirt as grass. After less than 30 years of existence, in a city that had tripled in size over that same span, Norte Del Rio was deemed expendable in light of community apathy and declining enrollment.

No one wanted to go there.

The school opened in 1954 as part of the exploding North Sacramento landscape that existed to support nearby McClellan Air Force Base—a civilian-employment powerhouse that is closed now as well. With the exception of former graduates, and sometimes not even those, it's hard to find anyone who has any fond memories of Norte Del Rio.

Even when it was open, Norte was Sacramento's forgotten high school. Bad or overly optimistic planning created an unwanted and unappealing appendage to a poorly managed inner-city school district with no money to spare. Norte lost academic-minded students to wealthier districts, to Catholic schools, or to wherever they could escape. As for athletics, Norte lost most of its stars to nearby Grant High School, which, although thought of as dangerous by the outside world, had a proud ethnic panache. Special academic programs such as aeronautics, classic Spanish architecture, and a rich sports history that could lay claim to launching the coaching careers of Milt Jackson, a longtime NFL and Pac-10 coach; and Rich Brooks, who went on to become head coach at Oregon, Kentucky, and later the St. Louis Rams, offered attractions that Norte couldn't muster. But Grant's coaches wouldn't have been successful without serious talent. Over the decades, Grant has produced numerous professional athletes, most recently Philadelphia Eagles wide receiver Donte Stallworth, Vikings running back Onterrio Smith, and 2001 Arena Football League MVP quarterback Aaron Garcia.

No insurmountable natural barriers—oceans or mountains—hinder Sacramento's expansion. With only the American and Sacramento rivers to straddle, the city's population perpetually surges in one direction or another. A new development here, approval to build there, all preceded by endless setbacks for environmentalists as the voracious sprawl gobbles up thousands of acres of wetlands wih each passing decade. Sacramento seems destined to become Northern California's version of L.A.

When Norte Del Rio first opened its doors, Sacramento's primary expansion was northward and showed no signs of slowing down. The booming Grant Union School District's plans for Norte were to endure the temporary structures, and then, over time, to add money and create special academic programs to equal those at Grant. Yet, that never happened. As far as the district and the city of Sacramento were concerned, Norte Del Rio was an unwanted stepchild. Nearly from the moment it opened its doors, it seemed insubstantial, if not rice-paper thin. The yearbooks, with black-and-white photographs and almost no captions, were colorless, slight, and bland. The school had no football stadium; and in fact, for the whole of its existence, Norte's football team had to play its games on the field of archrival Grant.

In the early '80s, Sacramento's insatiable northerly expansion slowed, and the city's housing boom spread east and south. Enrollment was on the decline, and Norte was hemorrhaging money. With no funds to rebuild and no wealthy alumni to push a reprieve, the school closed its doors forever in 1982 to little protest.

"The principal wouldn't communicate with the teachers, and the district's administrators refused to communicate with the principal," said longtime basketball coach, Carl Youngstrom, who taught at Norte for 25 years. "One day, we were just told it was over."

ONE MOMENT CHANGES EVERYTHING

Every dog has its day, so even wretched Norte Del Rio High School must have had a golden era—an era brought about by athletics. There must have been a time when scouts traveled from the nation's far reaches to join the denizens of Sacramento's rabid sports community to witness the wares of this school whose name translates literally to "north of the river."

Longtime Strawberry Manor residents, gray and too often haggard, remember when the area around Norte buzzed with pride. When, on game days, banners exalting the school's successes hung in windows and covered storefronts. After more than 25 years of futility, finally, Sacramento-area reporters had started to come to games at Norte, and the local papers had begun to sing the praises of the school's once-moribund athletic teams.

With no future ahead, little pride, and no sense of security in this war zone, when Norte Del Rio was finally thrust into the spotlight, it was because Don Rogers had taken the field. Don didn't come alone, either. He arrived as a sophomore sports and academic phenomenon in 1977, followed in 1979 by his younger brother, Reggie, a future NFL star who already stood 6-foot-4. And if that wasn't enough, a year later, their little sister, Jackie, enrolled. At 6-foot-2, Jackie was blessed with a rocket pitching arm and a soft baby hook—incredibly, she may have been the most gifted Rogers sibling of all.

In 2007, to reporters and residents who have lived in Sacramento for most of their lives, Norte Del Rio means one thing: The Rogers family. In the center of the least forgiving of American worlds—in the middle of a region of California that has managed to produce scores of professional athletes—the Rogers were so good they put a previously invisible high school on the map and managed to snatch the spotlight away from the area's traditional powers. In fact, the Rogers were so good, that few other memories of the Norte remain.

But that, of course, is also the sad part. Everything that Norte once was, whatever it was, is now gone. Celebrated or tainted as the Rogers' legacy is, the stars that played here, the people and events that put Norte into the news positively, the names that cause Heights residents to shake their heads and cry—they are all gone.

"It's sad, it hurts, and it's painful," said a man who runs a Strawberry Manor grocery store.

"They wasted themselves," 19-year-old Cloyd Ransom told the *Sacramento Bee*. "I looked to them for an example. A lot of teenagers did." He shakes his head. "They were such good athletes, you can't believe they would waste themselves like that. Why?"

The Rogers were a mixture of physical anomaly, human frailty, beauty, community spirit, and love of family—the rise and fall and the boom and bane of the all-or-nothing burden of urban life and poverty. But like the sorrow, the judgments come later. The should-haves and the would-haves of regret are plentiful, and are, unfortunately, too big a part of what remains. After decades of struggle, first for a school and then later for a family and a neighborhood, there was at least that one golden era of greatness.

When Don Rogers entered Norte in the tenth grade, the profile of the school was elevated immediately and then forever defined. The serious, dignified young man who would go on to make the honor roll every year, start at quarterback all three seasons, run hurdles with the state's best sprinters, brush the rim with his afro on follow-up jams, and touch the community with his humility and kindness was a walking, talking phenomenon. All that, and he was a doting son—a momma's boy, even—and by every account, the preternaturally heroic older brother.

F. Scott Fitzgerald once said, "Show me a hero, and I'll write you a tragedy." And there, in 1977, marked the appearance of the hero.

Don Lavert Rogers was a force of one. By examining the full-page tribute to him in Norte's 1980 yearbook—his senior year—perhaps one can begin to understand just how much one young man can matter. This early glimpse reveals the power of Don's influence, not only to his family but to his school and his neighborhood as well.

"Don was everyone's father, even mine."

ONE MOMENT CHANGES EVERYTHING

When Don Rogers entered Norte he was just over six feet tall, a little more than an inch shy of his adult height, and already sported his trademark crooked grin—not a smirk—but a grin that looked like one side of his face was frozen stiff in pleasant restraint. Well known for his junior high school achievements, there was no guarantee that his enrollment at Norte would have the impact it did, as many kids from sports-crazed Del Paso Heights enter Norte or Grant High with glittering reputations from watered-down Pop Warner leagues only to get cut from the JV team. Veteran high school coaches know that, too often, kids who star when they are young, those who are quick to develop, who arrive in high school with the biggest reputations, often disappoint when the other kids mature.

Not so with Don Rogers, however—Norte head basketball coach Carl Youngstrom remembers the first time he saw Don in person.

"I walked into the gym, and there was this young kid off shooting by himself," Youngstrom recalled. "He was dunking so easily—rims had no give in those days, and we couldn't afford new ones—so I was about to yell at him to stop. I was a purist, and up until that point, I was against dunking. Well, after watching Don take off from outside the key a few times, I have to admit, I wasn't against it any more."

Youngstrom estimates that, throughout his three-year high school career, Rogers slammed in games over 100 times.

"Typical sequence," says Dale Burney, a former four-sport star at rival Grant High, one-time AAU coach of Don and Reggie, and a man who spent part of his honeymoon visiting Don at UCLA the week before Rogers won MVP of the 1983 Rose Bowl. "Missed shot bounces high off the rim, and the other team's big men, a half-foot taller than Don, all go up for the board.

"But as the other players recede, Don just goes up and up and up, and he snags the ball and comes down with it in a crowd," Burney continued. "Everyone's slapping at him, but he's stronger, and no way is anyone getting that ball. Don gathers himself, jukes, dribbles once, and goes up and flushes it with two hands over a 6-

foot-7 forward who hasn't even had time to get back up off the ground."

Photographs of Don's unstoppable flights—there are no less than six photos of Rogers dunking in Norte Del Rio's 1980 yearbook—tangibly support Youngstrom and Burney's memories. Ball in one hand, arm stretched high above his head, Rogers is three feet off the floor and rearing back to throw down a jam as the defender, who having given up attempting to draw a charge, tries frantically to get out of the way.

Don is jumping completely over the other player, who has something original to tell his children that perhaps no one else can: "NFL star Don Rogers once jumped over me in a high school basketball game."

Of course, Don couldn't have been known just for basketball. From his junior season onward, he was the unquestioned leader and team captain of three varsity sports: football, basketball, and track, where he had times of 9.8 and 14.1 in the 100-yard dash and 120-yard high hurdles, respectively, making the California state finals in the high hurdles. And while he starred for Norte at the position he would play in college at UCLA, and in pros with the Cleveland Browns, free safety, Don was also Sacramento's premier option quarterback. Voted first-team All-City and elected to the Optimist All-Star football team as a senior, Don passed for 975 yards and eight touchdowns, including one strike that traveled 71 yards in the air, and rushed for 700 yards and four more scores—all for a team that had more than one starting lineman who tipped the scales somewhere *under* 150 pounds. Norte somehow managed to win six of ten games, but everyone affiliated with the program will readily admit that, without Don Rogers, Norte might not have won anything at all.

Don received numerous scholarship offers to play quarterback at the college level—but it was in basketball where he earned his greatest high school acclaim, leading Norte to an all-time school-best 24-4 record, earning a coveted and illustrious spot on the All-Northern California Basketball Team. He was then voted to play in

ONE MOMENT CHANGES EVERYTHING

Sacramento's annual Optimist All-Star Basketball game, where he won the slam-dunk contest and was the game's MVP.

A prolific scorer who created his own points, Don averaged 21.2 points per game to rank fifth in the Sacramento Section, which is comprised of roughly 100 high schools. Perhaps more remarkably, as a 6-foot-2 forward who was often matched against players six or seven inches taller, he averaged 14 rebounds per game, which was also good for fifth place in the section. No other player managed to rank in the top 15 in two categories. Sixty points and 39 rebounds were Rogers' two-game totals from a weekend tournament his senior year. Points and rebound totals of 36 and 15, 22-21, 25-10, and 33-14 were his lines for two weeks' worth of games later that same season.

Taken out of context, those random numbers mean little. Consider reconciling them as totals achieved in 32-minute contests, against teams with slowdown offenses and zone-gimmick defenses, without a three-point line or shot clock, and with the constant probability that anytime you touched an opponent, a whistle would blow. Consider all of that, and one begins to comprehend the outrageous athletic ability that is necessary for a 6-foot-2 forward to dominate games so thoroughly.

Don's outstanding performances on the court, as well on the track and football field, often generated headlines. Yet, as any press agent will say, despite talent, it helps to be imbued with a little "fluky" good fortune once in a while. Surnames that lend themselves to easy rhyme or association to other famous people, places, or events make for good copy, and Don was no exception. There was this charming little "wink," a connection between Don and his high school that made it seem as if Rogers was made for Norte, and Norte was made for Don. Norte Del Rio High's mascot was—and it's probably nothing more than a coincidence—The Don.

The Norte Del Rio Dons.

The prodigiously talented eldest Rogers child was motivated by more than catchy headlines or fame, though. In fact, most people who knew him agree that he didn't care about headlines at all. Even early on, he was single-minded about success. He rarely attended school dances or went to parties, instead electing to stay home and study after practice and games. He seemed to be on a quest to thrive—or to escape.

"It was their only way out," said Loretha, referring to her children's connection to studies and sports.

Off the court and field, Don was a gentleman. "It was my mom who taught me to be polite," he once told *The Los Angeles Times*. He held doors open for women, and always said, "yes, ma'am," and "please" and "thank you."

But during games Don transformed into an unparalleled competitor, a driven, intense athlete with only one thing in mind: winning.

"The best focus of any athlete I've ever seen," said basketball coach, Carl Youngstrom. "He wanted very much to be successful."

Don's life at home was loving, but impoverished and perhaps a bit schizophrenic. It's unclear whether he ever knew his real father, but everyone in The Heights knew Don's mother, Loretha, very well. She was six feet tall, proud, and regretted not having gotten a formal education—something her pregnancy with Don interrupted. Just as important were the values and sense of urgency she ingrained in her family, and it's worth noting that the Rogers matriarch was raised in a segregated Arkansas.

While Martin Luther King Jr. was being sentenced to four months of hard labor for merely sitting at the whites-only lunch counter in an otherwise empty Atlanta diner, Loretha was living in an even more restrictive and dangerous part of the country: Texarkana, Arkansas.

The scars created by years of racial discrimination—and the pain that was left in its wake—never healed for Loretha. This was, of course, government-mandated discrimination. While intervention by U.S. Attorney General Bobby Kennedy was necessary to secure King's release from jail, places like Texarkana, which are far less visible, less cosmopolitan than Atlanta were filled with blacks that became intrinsically aware of the universal need to protect their families at all costs. Because of laws that enforced school segregation in Arkansas until 1957—and other laws that encouraged and emboldened those who chose violent means to confront the issue—family ties were all that minority citizens living the South had.

To escape the life she'd known and to keep her child from having to live under the humiliation of oppression and the paranoia inherent to her situation, with Don just a baby and without money or assurances, Loretha and her sister bravely boarded a train and headed west to California.

Certainly, this wasn't the only time that Loretha put her children first. Later, after the precipitous rise and devastating collapse of her family, when nothing except their glorious past was left to defend, she would be called upon time and again to answer for the tragedies that had befallen her clan. While Loretha's reputation around Strawberry Manor differed from person to person—some saw her as combative, but most saw her as a passionately protective mother—her sense of right and wrong and the chip placed upon her shoulder by her childhood, was often evidenced by her actions around the community. When Loretha saw that most of Norte Del Rio's cheerleaders were Hispanic and not black, she went down to the school and complained. And in 1982, when Grant Union School District officials announced that Norte Del Rio would be closing its doors, it was Loretha who went down to the office and lodged a protest. All along, there were other, more pressing worries for Loretha—not only for her children's safety in Strawberry Manor, but because, sometimes, the family didn't have enough to eat.

"They were very poor," said Youngstrom. "They lived in a tiny house. I think all the kids shared one room."

Don may or may not have ever met his real father, but Reggie and Jackie knew their father, Joe Henry, quite well.

Joe Henry Rogers and Loretha had been separated for years before divorcing in 1980. Joe had gone to Grant High School, and while Loretha's pregnancy with Don back in Arkansas had forced her to turn down an offer to play basketball at prestigious all-black Grambling State University in Louisiana, Joe reportedly was an average athlete. A likeable, kind man, as an adult, Joe Rogers held jobs as a busboy, an airport Sky Cap, a laundry worker, a security guard, and a garbage collector. He also, reportedly, liked to imbibe.

"He came to games after he'd been drinking. He would be up in the stands, and it was obvious," said Youngstrom. "During time outs, first Don and later Reggie, you could see them glancing up. They couldn't help but notice him. Everyone knew."

A single mother in Strawberry Manor, a well-meaning father who was proud of his kids, not enough to eat—everyone knew.

Despite the hardships, in 1980, Don was unquestionably Sacramento's biggest sports star, and Loretha no doubt was filled with pride about her son's accomplishments. It was also readily apparent, to those in and around Del Paso Heights, that Reggie and Jackie were destined for similar greatness as well.

For Don, as well as for his siblings, high school stardom was only just the beginning of their rise to fame, their starting point. Along with the stardom, however, came headlines and increased visibility. And in the case of one of the siblings, the additional focus led to questions about character. Even as an ultra-talented high school football and basketball player, there were whispers about Reggie, some of which resulted from a curious decision he made during his sophomore year.

As a senior, Don earned every individual honor that was available to him in and around Sacramento. What, though, would have made his high school legacy greater still, and at the same time, kept whispers about his brother from surfacing in the first place? Oddly enough, winning a California state high school basketball championship.

In assessing his Sacramento Delta League champions, a team that advanced to the second round of the section playoffs, head coach Carl Youngstrom said: "We had great shooters, and Don was all over the place and impossible to stop. But what we needed to go all the way to the state finals was one more really good player. Someone with size, and a little more height."

Where was a high school with a shrinking enrollment going to get this height?

ONE MOMENT CHANGES EVERYTHING

"There was this extremely talented sophomore on the junior varsity. One of the two best players we ever had at Norte. He would have been the perfect fit for our team. He was a 6-foot-6 scoring and rebounding machine. He actually began the year on the varsity, but he suddenly decided he wanted to play with the JVs, instead. Don and I pleaded with him to stay up and help us, but he refused."

Refused to play varsity? Don's younger brother, Reggie?

When one learns just how far Reggie Rogers' talent would take him, that he refused the opportunity to play varsity with his brother his sophomore year is a strange addendum indeed.

"The three of us met early in the season, with Don and I trying to persuade Reggie to stay. I had the sense it had to be done gently. I told Reggie he could start games or come off the bench. Any role that made him feel comfortable. This is Del Paso Heights—sports are everything—and I never, before or after, had to offer that for a player.

"But Reggie wouldn't budge. And he wouldn't say why. He just insisted. Later that week, I thought I'd ask Don about it one last time. There's no doubt in my mind that Reggie's decision concerned Don. But nevertheless, Don looked me right in the eye and told me, man to man, 'It's done, Coach. It's over. He's not coming back.'"

The pressure on talented teenagers who play sports, especially kids with size-16 sneakers, is too randomly and too callously applied by coaches, parents, and fans: People that want to win games. Complicating things is the fact that bigger kids are just thought to be naturally tougher, thicker-skinned, and able to "take it." The misperception is that size equals emotional maturity.

Don was a great player as a sophomore, averaging 24 points a game for the JVs. But varsity is where the meaningful games are played, and once Don starred there, his reputation began to grow right along with Norte's. When Don was a senior, Reggie was a sophomore and forced into the role of following in his older brother's footsteps. The downside of Don's success was that people felt compelled to expect the exact same things of Reggie.

THE ALL-AMERICA TRAGEDY OF DON ROGERS

Don seems to have understood, though—more than most adults, anyway—that he and his brother were built differently. Taking a cue from Loretha, throughout their lives the older brother came to the younger brother's aid in scrapes, fights, and on the playing fields—where he always made certain that the two were on the same team. Reggie may have sometimes cruised through games, but true to his nature, Don remained Reggie's biggest supporter. During later interviews, he would often refer to his brother, and their sister, Jackie, as inspirations. By all accounts, Don was as much a father to his younger brother and sister as he was a sibling.

In regard to the early differences between Don and Reggie, author George Thomas Clark, a writer and news correspondent who spent four years covering area high school sports for the *Sacramento Bee*, wrote in April 2005 about his recollections of covering the Rogers brothers.

Clark first met Don in 1978 when the reporter had come to Norte to interview local track star Roy Mosley. The 16-year-old Rogers walked up and politely introduced himself.

After a few minutes' conversation, for the only time in his career as a journalist, Clark was compelled to give out his telephone number to a "high school kid." The correspondent saw something in Rogers, saying, "He was a charming guy that people instinctively liked and trusted." He wanted Don to keep in touch.

Two years after their initial meeting, Clark was assigned to cover Norte's basketball game against the Jesuit High Marauders, a league rival and a private, boys-only Catholic school located in the upscale Sacramento suburb of Carmichael, near the American River. The governor's mansion is just a few blocks away.

Jesuit is a California sports and academic power that, in both 1993 and 1994, advanced all the way to the state Division I basketball championship game—losing both times. The school has produced numerous college players in several sports, most notably former New York Jets quarterback Ken O'Brien, and Olympic gold-medal swimmer Jeff Float.

ONE MOMENT CHANGES EVERYTHING

Clark obviously witnessed something extraordinary that night in the Jesuit gym, something that statistics alone could never define. The morning after the game, Clark's column began, "The Rogers brothers were unleashed on Jesuit High School Tuesday night, and the Marauders are probably still flinching."

In an April 2005 recap of the evening written almost 27 years later entitled, "The Rogers Brothers—Triumph and Tragedy," Clark writes:

> I'd arrived a little earlier than usual so I could watch a good chunk of the junior-varsity game featuring Donald's sophomore brother, 6-foot-6 Reggie. As I approached the scorer's table, people shouted to me, "Hey, Reggie had 24 points in the first quarter, and he scored the team's first 33 points." ...
>
> Reggie Rogers cooled off in the third quarter, but poured in 16 points in the final and finished with 59 and a victory. Next, in the main event, Donald scored 36. It was an exhilarating evening. But one thing troubled me: why wasn't Reggie Rogers playing varsity, where he belonged? I asked the Norte coach and he said during preseason practice Reggie had demanded to be sent down to the JVs. ...

Clark finished by declaring, "Something in his [Reggie's] makeup compelled him to avoid the appropriate athletic challenges and, instead, dominate much smaller and weaker players."

Written so many years after that spectacular night of promise, even after the still-to-come tragedies had all played out, this observation, made by a writer who was himself a star high school athlete, was profound for two reasons. One, because of his background, Clark appreciated the greatness of such dominance; and two, he was struck, even troubled, by the fact that this 16-year-old *man* chose to play against boys. When the final legacy and chapter of Reggie Rogers' life is complete, and all the opinions and pens are laid down, Clark may well have asked the one question that is the most impossible to answer: Why wasn't Reggie where he belonged?

But as frustrated as people both inside and outside the Rogers' circle must have been at Reggie's refusal to engage the challenges available to him, the questions and confusion don't begin to end there.

"I knew Don meant it (that Reggie's decision to play JV was final) and I tried to respect his position," Norte coach Youngstrom added. "We got on with it and had a great year. But once the JV season was complete, and we made the T.O.C., we still desperately needed size, so I asked Reggie if he would finish the season with us. I was as surprised as anyone when he agreed."

A recurring Reggie theme was introduced clearly on a public stage for the first time. Ever the enigma, opinions of the young Reggie vary. In some circles, he was applauded for going his own way; while other people, frustrated area fans, reporters, students, and varsity teammates in particular, viewed him with disgust for taking the easy way out to star against lesser competition. But there's no denying that his brother, Don, and the entire varsity team, lightning fast but small, needed Reggie's size and physical strength to make an otherwise-good season spectacular.

In the section playoff game, because of foul trouble—he had three in the first quarter alone—Reggie's playing time was limited, but he still managed to score eight points and block two shots as Norte lost a nail-biter to end the year.

Both of Norte's coaches, Youngstrom and Burney, agree that, had Reggie played with the varsity for the entire season, nothing would have been beyond the team's grasp—including a state title. But coaches and fans are like that, and seasons are often viewed in the context of that final loss, and why it should never have occurred.

Then again, knowing what came later for Reggie, there were never any guarantees.

Leaders and champions such as Don Rogers are made not merely of confidence or raw talent, which are somewhat common, but more importantly, winners are born of the courage to risk

ONE MOMENT CHANGES EVERYTHING

failure. Talent in the form of jumping ability and precise timing may earn a good athlete more than his share of rebounds, but only talent infused with fortitude and toughness can turn a 6-foot-2 jumping jack like Don Rogers into one of the most prolific rebounders in the history of California.

It was apparent early on to those who knew them that Don and Reggie, both literally and figuratively, were born of different fathers. The two didn't look or act alike. And though they were both singularly gifted athletes, as was Jackie, even their physical talents were profoundly disparate, as Don relied on agility and speed while Reggie was larger and more powerful.

But how different can two brothers be? And why would Reggie refuse to play varsity?

Over time, the consensus on Reggie has adopted the opinion that he simply wilts under pressure or stress of any kind. Yet, going down to play on the JV, Reggie was accepting that he would be the focal point of the team. There's certainly pressure in that. Playing with his brother would have absorbed much of the glare as well, allowing Reggie to test his abilities while also helping the varsity, which, under the circumstances, would have been the popular thing to do.

Many people in America see talent as a community property that owes the public its integrity. The public gets upset when a person more gifted than they are doesn't behave as they think he or she should. And the public can become downright indignant when talent becomes corrupted by lust or avarice or fame. But it's all quite possible that Reggie was merely being young, self-centered, and stubborn, and simply didn't think his decision through clearly.

Yet one wonders how he could face Don each morning at the breakfast table. Considering what is known about Don, he would probably have made it easy on his brother. By some accounts, Don was always the favored son. Loretha deferred to him early and often, which hastened his maturity, but also may have increased his already profound stress and, possibly, even caused guilt. People learn to deal with those emotional assailants in their own ways. But Don was highly intelligent, even sensitive and instinctive. He may well have realized he was favored and done anything he could to assuage the inequity—perhaps even going overboard to protect his younger brother by deferring to him.

Obviously, Reggie stayed on the JV team in order to play against the younger, lesser competition, and thus be the star of the team. There's nothing criminal about that. Reggie was easily the best sophomore in Sacramento—an absolutely dominant player—and just as his brother did, he led his team in points and rebounds. Yet, when George Clark's assessment regarding Reggie's makeup is combined with the opinion of Norte's varsity basketball coach, a pattern is unveiled, something that appeals to different people in and around the Rogers camp for reasons as varied as the brothers themselves.

In his interview for this book, Youngstrom said something about Reggie that would keep most self-respecting athletes awake at night. In light of future events, it's a statement that remains impossible to ignore. "The entire time I knew him," said Youngstrom, "Reggie always looked for the easy way out."

Despite all the negativity orbiting the world of sports—a force produced mostly by its own inhabitants—the truly great moments are still deified as makers of men (and women). Short of the unfathomable, disturbing experiences of war, or even the dangers of the toughest streets, sports do indeed provide opportunities for young people to excel and rise above their circumstances. Reggie's refusal to play varsity represents a missed opportunity and an early and unfortunate example of a troubled young man. Had he been pushed early on or possessed more discipline, he might have never created the tragic events that would startle a nation.

Instead, Reggie showed, or was allowed to show, just how desperate he was to avoid pressure, just how much he needed to take the easy way out, and indeed, how absolutely determined he was to escape his brother's immense shadow. In and of themselves, none of these is an unforgivable sin or even unusual behavior for a teen. At the time, if Don had had not been so resolutely admired for his will and leadership, this would not be nearly as noteworthy.

ONE MOMENT CHANGES EVERYTHING

However, in reviewing Clark's evaluation, one can only guess whether or not the middle Rogers child was possessed by the desire, or worse, the need to beat up on lesser competition. The need to humiliate is not a characteristic of a healthy soul, and even in the most charitable of appraisals, at best, reveals the core values of a bully. But intense, unrelenting pressure befalls a kid when a sibling is a beloved superstar, and only two years older, as well. And there's Joe Henry, Reggie's father, who hardly seems a role model.

Poverty and the apparent inequity of a mother's affection would ingrain issues that threaten to harm children, even those born into idyllic homes. From this school of thought, despite his prodigious talent, the stars were never aligned in favor of Reggie Rogers. In the teenage sports world, superlatives are easy to come by—just ask any wide-eyed parent whose child scores ten points for the freshman basketball team. Each year, millions of kids play high school football and basketball; and the number of players who garner awards, see their names in the newspaper, or make all-star or all-tournament teams is staggering. Throw in individual sports, and Extreme Sports, and everyone gets a trophy just for falling down.

So how does one differentiate Don Rogers from myriad other stars at the high school level, and how well did Reggie and Jackie perform once their brother went away to UCLA? One perspective takes the lens of what will happen later. To be sure, only a couple of athletes have accomplished anything comparable to what Don Rogers did at UCLA. Yet, while Don paved the way for his siblings, he also greased the skids of the immense burden of comparison. Don used a machete to hack his way out of the jungle, with his siblings fast on his trail—but jungle trails invariably become overgrown with obstructions and hangers-on, especially in a place like Strawberry Manor.

Don was not only the first from his family, he was the greatest from his school and arguably the best ever from a neighborhood that was soon to become known as a national recruiting hotbed for athletic talent. Don wasn't the very first to receive an elite scholarship from his neighborhood, but he would be the most celebrated and well known.

THE ALL-AMERICA TRAGEDY OF DON ROGERS

Throughout the 1980s, UCLA was a national power in football and a perennial top-ten team in the Associated Press weekly poll. So when head coach Terry Donahue began repeating to anyone who would listen that he intended to mold Don into the next great Bruin safety, a position manned at the time by the All-American—and future Hall of Famer—Kenny Easley, several cynics suddenly arose amongst his former fans in the neighborhood. For apparently no reason other than envy, some people began to predict that Don would fail at the next level.

When Don didn't fail, though—when, in fact, he thrived—perhaps those same cynics instead turned their jealousy toward the next in the Rogers' line, diverting Reggie from the well-paved path that Don had created.

Regardless of Reggie's sophomoric decision not to play varsity basketball at Norte, Don, Reggie, and Jackie's ascent to stardom was only just beginning. The Rogers' combined athletic accomplishments would soon equal or exceed those of any siblings in California history—and no one, except for perhaps the Rogers themselves, could stand in the way of that.

2

Don had graduated and moved on to UCLA, but Reggie was in his junior year at Norte, where their sister, Jackie, had entered as a sophomore. The school's once-overlooked profile was now red hot with talent and athletic spectacle. Expectations had risen, and people around town were watching closely.

Reggie was nearing his adult height of 6-foot-6, but his broad shoulders and wingspan approached 7 feet, and his build was a lean 210 pounds. On the high school football fields of the early 1980s, before year-round training and the common use of supplements and steroids, players over 200 pounds were not all that common. An average high school team might boast two or three 200-pounders at best—so Reggie, although renowned more for his "speed" rush from the outside than his pure strength, had a size advantage over most competitors. On the way to becoming a complete player, Reggie played tight end as well, becoming a very good blocker and receiver.

Yet, he still had a troubling reputation for sitting out plays on both sides of the ball.

With Reggie playing varsity then, Norte's football team, which had gone from laughingstock to league-title contender during Don's tenure, regressed to something less than average. Although they were still far better than before Don, when one or two wins per season was considered the norm, a blazing-fast, super-smart option quarterback like Don is a bigger asset to any team than a comparably talented defensive lineman. Don's impact on the game, and his absence thereof, reverberated during each play from scrimmage.

Or perhaps, in light of Reggie's failure to be elected a full-time captain for the football or basketball team, Don's distinguished leadership abilities had left the biggest void at Norte. "Don was very serious, but Reggie was more of a character," said a former coach.

Reggie inherited undisputed stardom on both teams, but the success of high school sports teams, even more than at the college level, depends on good ball-handlers, quarterbacks, leaders, and distributors. As a post player and a defensive lineman, Reggie could be double- or even triple-teamed in either sport, allowing teams to attack other places on the court or field. Being the focus of the other team, though, did not keep Reggie from achieving that stardom.

Like his older brother, Reggie loved to dunk and could do so with absolute ease. Reggie wasn't merely tall—his astounding leaping ability augmented his size even more. Reggie once showed up at a Norte Del Rio track meet and, without a warm-up, high-jumped six feet, five inches. But unlike Don, when he dunked, Reggie tried to tear down the rim with each slam. He seemed to have something to prove and often played out of control, even angry, constantly accumulating unnecessary fouls, which led to several foul-out disqualifications—a habit that would follow him into college. (For his part, Don never fouled out of a single high school game.)

Yet, as his star rose, and his reputation grew, Reggie had to contend with something that had never been an issue for his older brother. Unlike Don, the towering Reggie found himself the target of opposing fans. "People called me nigger all the time," Reggie recently said, "even kids."

In terms of high school pressure, Reggie's lowest moments emotionally came against Norte's league rival, the mostly white Jesuit High. Besides being an athletic powerhouse—Jesuit would spend much of 2007 amongst the nation's top-25 teams by

CNNSI—the school incubates future Ivy League and Stanford students.

With the advent of ESPN, the frenzied behavior of "amped-up" student bodies was being broadcast nationwide by the mid-1980s. Disparaging chants, dizzying gyrations, card tricks—all performed at high-decibel levels—helped to create an atmosphere of energy and bedlam at college games that was absent from professional sports contests.

Even before ESPN set the uniform standard for fan exuberance, though, Jesuit High School had already become Sacramento's elite. An overflow crowd in the large Jesuit gymnasium—with the knees of fans "unintentionally" jabbing into the backs of visiting team players—was every bit as intimidating and distracting to a group of 17-year-old high school basketball players as any Atlantic Coast Conference arena.

The Jesuit High School boys, whose parents paid several thousand dollars a year in tuition, had not forgotten that Reggie dropped 33 straight points on their JV team a year earlier. In January of 1981, perhaps harking back to Don's varsity heroics, they were determined to swing the odds into their favor by any means necessary.

Commencing days before the actual game, the entire Jesuit High campus conspired, with unbridled excitement, to harass Reggie. Boys painted their faces blood red and wore military fatigues to face down Reggie, who, upon Don's graduation, had become Sacramento's biggest sports star.

Jesuit team members were just as innovative as their student body. When opponents had breakaways, Jesuit players—even those farthest away from the play—would proceed to belly-ski across the wood floor like penguins sliding on a sheet of ice at Sea World. In the annals of high school sports history, the action was every bit as odd as it was original.

The goal, it seemed, was to incite the student body to ever-greater levels of harassment and frenzy, to collect floor burns, to discombobulate opponents. While the Jesuit fans loved it, Norte's players felt engaged in a battle of wills with a team full of crazies.

ONE MOMENT CHANGES EVERYTHING

Norte was *the* big game for Jesuit, which finished just behind the Dons in each of the previous two seasons. The Jesuit fans were determined to be part of the show and affect the outcome of the game. They blew whistles, threw objects, cracked blocks of wood together, and shrieked in the ears of the Norte players. Several times, fans surged forward so that students fell into the Norte bench and onto the playing floor into a heap.

Complaints from Norte did little but escalate the fury. The bleachers and court shook so violently that Norte coach Carl Youngstrom couldn't use his chalkboard to diagram plays. With opposing fans only a few feet away, Youngstrom's instructions to his players would've gone unheard anyway.

While the student body's goal may have been a Jesuit win, they reserved their most poignant vitriolic energies for Reggie. During a timeout, whenever he would come to the bench, the students would point at him, jabbing their fingers, literally, within inches of his face and the back of his head. When Reggie collected a third foul early in the second quarter, instead of cheering for the rest of the game, the fans chanted:

"REG-GIE SUCKS! REG-GIE SUCKS! REG-GIE SUCKS!"

Though this behavior is considered good fun in 2007, the sports landscape in 1981 had featured nothing like it. What Reggie perceived as hatred aimed specifically at him, was indeed unsettling. He tried to focus on the game, but found it nearly impossible to block out the chanting. When he fouled out in the fourth quarter, rather than endure the taunts, Youngstrom excused his star. Beneath personal jeers that undoubtedly would incite a reaction from a professional athlete, Reggie, head bowed, made his way to the Norte locker room.

Reggie would constantly tell friends, reporters, and family members that he just wanted to play basketball. "Why were they doing this?" he wondered. He was—figuratively as well as literally—the biggest star in Sacramento, but he truly could not comprehend why opposing fans were targeting him. Was it merely his race? The Jesuit brand of mockery set a precedent for

Sacramento-area high school sports. Some saw it as the first sign of a coming apocalypse, and the media latched onto enough people's outrage at such behavior, receiving several letters of protest against such behavior.

While his play was consistently sterling, things only got worse for Reggie as his high school career continued.

Norte's schedule included several games against predominately white schools. While the progressive administrations, fans, and parents in and around Sacramento would never have tolerated a student body calling out an opposing player based on race, Norte's non-conference schedule took the heavily minority school to away games in small communities outside the city—small towns with few black faces, where tolerance for bigotry was menacingly high. In such a place, Reggie's much-anticipated senior season of football came to an abrupt and violent end on a farm-town football field 50 miles northwest of Sacramento.

As the third game of the 1981 season approached, Reggie already had been honored as a member of at least one preseason All-America team as a defensive lineman. While this recognition may have given credence to the notion that Reggie benefited from his older brother's shadow, the distinction was a double-edged sword. Outsiders dissected unearned accolades with consternation, but Reggie saw the honors as disadvantages he neither wanted nor needed.

Reggie was already a major prep star in California, not in the least because his brother was starting free safety for nationally ranked UCLA. Small-town powers such as Winters High School, desperate for rays of refracted fame, craved urban publicity; and beating Norte—and Reggie Rogers—was their chance to attract a piece of the spotlight.

If, in 30 years' time, Winters High School had even one player receive a sports scholarship to a major university, the town probably would've named a street after him. So when someone such as Reggie Rogers came to Winters, everyone—every player, every fan, the school itself, *everyone*—found their biggest opportunity to shine.

ONE MOMENT CHANGES EVERYTHING

To most high school athletes, facing a star of Reggie Rogers' caliber—a future first-round NFL draft pick—is the most significant moment of their athletic lives, something they can someday tell their children. Furthermore, such a game, one that contains players from such disparate backgrounds, is the essence of competition. In its best light, the contest should have been lauded as an opportunity for the two student bodies to expand their worlds and grow.

So how did it all go so violently wrong?

If an event such as the one that follows were to occur today—with a star like Reggie Rogers at its epicenter—a dozen handheld cameras, camera phones, and probably news crews would've been on hand to ensure the events were replayed nonstop on ESPN.

Then again, if it happened today, there would probably be gunfire.

Although prior to the explosion of inner-city gangs and before the proliferation of cable television—both of which would've worsened the scene—what transpired was ugly. Very little media attended the game, and security and police were slow to arrive. What's worse, they were indecisive once they did arrive; or, perhaps, less indecisive as they were feigning confusion. At the center of everything were the children, friends, and neighbors of the Winters police department, which, according to dozens of eyewitnesses, seemed less than anxious to control the situation.

Happening too late that Friday night, too far from the city to make the morning papers, the incident instead earned a vague, static front-page recap that raised more questions than it answered. Over the weekend, school administrators, covering for their small district, complemented by agenda-laced, second-hand accounts of eyewitnesses, further diluted the story with the ever-present "they started it" mentality.

No one wanted to accept responsibility.

When Norte coaches scheduled a game against Winters High School for late September 1981, they probably considered earning an easy win against a little-known school from the sticks, thought about giving the inner-city Norte players a chance to see some of the countryside that surrounded their hometown. For the Winters High School football team, though, the game was the only one that mattered. The school was a little-known Division III power that was nearly impossible to find on a map. The fact that Don Rogers—who had played for UCLA on television the previous weekend—and his brother Reggie had already put Norte on a different kind of map only added to the excitement.

Articles in the Winters paper detailed the exploits of the now 6-foot-6, 225-pound Reggie Rogers, printing an almost unbelievable list of the prestigious universities that were recruiting him for both football and basketball. The Winters players knew that this was their chance to make a name for themselves, but had the good folks of the tiny town ever seen anything like Reggie Rogers?

Winters was then a hamlet of about 1,000 people, most of whom brought along their cousins and jammed into the bleachers of the stadium for their team's most anticipated game in years. Fans were encouraged to bring their cowbells and yell. The Winters JVs utilized their triple-option attack to perfection, running Norte's sophomores off the field. The fans were out in force, vocal and hostile, and ticket sales for the sold-out game halted at halftime of the JV contest. Townspeople who were unable to get tickets lined the cyclone fence surrounding the stadium. Cars added to the bedlam by passing on Main Street and honking.

The first two quarters of the varsity game were close, physical, and hard fought. Complaints came from the Norte sideline—Winters was out for blood, and their players were yelling "Nigger!" as they made tackles.

An ominous event occurred at halftime. Breaking with tradition, Norte's JV coaches didn't wait until the varsity game was over to put their players on the team bus and drive back to Sacramento. Later, they would tell investigators that they left early because the home crowd had been directing racial slurs and threats in their direction.

During the game, in violation of rules, some home team fans began to line the end zones. When a pass intended for Norte receivers was overthrown, Dons had to force their way through the adults to get back on the field. Norte head coach Dave Pope asked the officials to move the crowd back. They complied, but this seemed to enrage the spectators, who brazenly began to direct racial epithets at Norte players.

Everyone could hear them.

Penalties, shoving matches, and trash talk marred the fourth quarter. The referees brought the players together at midfield and told them that the remainder of the game would be cancelled if the fighting and name-calling didn't end immediately. After the break, things calmed down, and Winters High emerged with a surprisingly easy 13-0 victory—but that was just the beginning.

"In retrospect, we shouldn't have allowed the teams to gather for the postgame handshake," said a Winters city official. A punch was thrown—no one knows by whom—and a fight broke out. In a flash, over 400 adults stormed the field. Weapons appeared, and helmets went flying as the spectators attacked the Norte players.

Of course, Loretha Rogers was there, and after proudly watching Reggie record a couple of sacks, she was ready to put him in the car and take him back to Sacramento. She was left watching the melee that ensued, though, until Reggie suddenly disappeared from view. In a flash, she sprinted down the stadium steps, hurdled the guardrail, and joined the fray.

"Grown men were carrying bats and chains," she would later say.

It took Loretha several minutes to locate Reggie. He was on the ground, seriously injured. Three men, at least one of which held a metal pipe in his hands, were jumping around, taunting her son as he lay in a daze. Loretha got between Reggie and the men. They moved in menacingly, but then retreated when players from Winters interceded.

Seventeen-year-old Reggie Rogers had a shattered right arm and internal injuries.

The next morning, the two Sacramento newspapers had nearly identical headlines that read: "Norte Player Hurt in Fight" and "Norte Del Rio Player Hurt". Watchmen with language skills, whose job is simply to report the facts of big stories as accurately and succinctly as possible, probably wrote those articles late at night. Not until Monday morning did *Sacramento Union* and *Bee* staff writers have the opportunity to thoroughly investigate the incident, and—for what probably seemed like the 1,000th time in the past couple years alone—create a headline with the name "Rogers" in bold print.

Only this was the family's very first headline with an unhappy ending. Unfortunately, it wouldn't be the last.

As for Reggie, he would recover, but his senior season of football was over after only three games—so much for the All-America team. Because of his injuries, however, both USC and Ohio State temporarily backed off from recruiting him for football. It didn't matter. The day after the brawl, Reggie made a major decision: he was tired of football, and probably tired of comparisons to his brother. Henceforth, he would focus only on basketball.

Still, most college football coaches continued to salivate over Reggie's unique combination of size, power, and speed. Most experts were certain he would have no difficulty playing both sports at the next level. Football recruiters were knocking on his door and calling his house late into the night. While besides Ohio State and USC, Reggie continued to be courted for football by several elite football colleges, his grades were not nearly as high as Don's, so he would not follow his brother to an academically discerning UCLA.

While Don had been a dominant player in both football and basketball, as a 6-foot-2 forward, little doubt surrounded which sport he would pursue at the collegiate level. The only question had been, "What position would he play?" Besides, Don, in some ways, was a finished physical product, while Reggie offered loads of potential to add strength and put on size.

Reggie, though, never really controlled football games the way Don had—or worse, the way everyone expected he should. To make matters more complicated, football was not Reggie's true passion. Deep down, he only wanted to play basketball, and he wanted to play it in the NBA. His injury at Winters High had been the final straw that—for the time being, at least—erased any passion he had for football.

The investigation into the Winters riot would last for weeks; but in the end, no arrests were made. Loretha had contacted the local police, the FBI, both school boards, and the Sacramento-area media, but to no avail.

It was, however, the advent of something new. The Rogers family had received its first real taste of negative fame, and reporters called at all hours to ask Reggie uncomfortable and sometimes misleading questions. "It was about race," Loretha said at the time. She complained to the media that the Winters police disregarded her story, filed a grossly incomplete report, made no effort to find the men who had attacked her son or other Norte players.

Yet, within the attack's circumstances remains the microcosm of Reggie Rogers himself. He was a star target, and a target because he was a star; because he was a black star; because he was a man amongst boys. Coincidence? Reggie Rogers did not deserve what happened at Winters, and it's safe to say that he didn't instigate the brawl or fuel the throng's ire. Contrarily, he was apparently innocent and simply a case of wrong person, wrong place, wrong time.

Despite his spartan upbringing, Reggie had the world at his feet—but he also had a target on his back, and one that he himself did not place there. The question was: Would Reggie Rogers do enough in his future to remove himself from that very same hit list?

Time would tell.

No one but the Winters police department truly knows how diligently they pursued an investigation. They couldn't have had much else, if anything, to do. To Loretha, however, what happened in Winters must have been a terrifying reminder of the life that she had to believe was left in the Deep South.

Safety is relative, though. The type of threats that, in 1981, still lurked in small towns such as Winters would indeed lessen over time. Despite Loretha's concerns, back home—in what was supposed to be one of the most dangerous of California neighborhoods—the Rogers family would be safe with their lean matriarch at the helm.

At least for now.

With Reggie injured and shelved for the remainder of football season—as well as the beginning of his senior basketball season—much of Del Paso Heights turned its attention to a sport that had traditionally garnered very little respect locally. As it had under Don's watch, Norte would continue to challenge rival Grant for neighborhood, even Sacramento sports supremacy, but in new and different ways.

Norte was becoming a rising power in girls basketball. For the first time ever, both Norte and Grant high schools saw their teams ranked in the top-five of Northern California.

Jackie Rogers was the reason.

3

Grant had always been a girls' basketball power. Even though nationwide many people lacked a connection to female sports; in places like Del Paso Heights, championship girls teams had managed to cultivate followings.

Female squads like those at Norte, though, lacked support universally. Often understaffed and always underfunded, attracting coaches was even less a problem than attracting girls. Contrasted to the boys' squad, which had to cut over 50 players just to get down to a 12-man roster, Norte had just eight girls come out for their team before Jackie arrived.

Just as Don's arrival altered Norte's fortunes, Jackie's enrollment spotlighted the girls' programs. While Reggie's accomplishments continued to enhance and further the Rogers' legacy, Jackie's entrance cemented the perception that Norte was a place to be.

Jackie Rogers was a rare talent who was fun to watch because she made dominance look so effortless. While she certainly hated to lose and wanted to win as badly as anyone—crying after tough losses—she often smiled on the court, and could be seen congratulating opponents for good plays, almost to a fault. She never complained about calls that didn't go her way.

Battling several other girls for a loose ball that no one could seem to handle, she once asked, in a detached voice, "Doesn't anybody want this thing?" Once the ball was finally controlled, players from both sides, as well as the referees, broke out in laughter.

ONE MOMENT CHANGES EVERYTHING

To this day, some sportswriters believe that Jackie Rogers is the most gifted athlete in Sacramento history. The consensus claims she was every bit as talented as her older brothers, which places her in contention for the city's best ever by expert opinion.

One of the most beautiful girls in the neighborhood, by her junior year Jackie had already reached her adult height of over 6 feet. She was lithe and graceful with long limbs, and she moved with a smooth, confident glide, a soft voice, and large brown eyes. If Don was the natural leader, the captain calling alignments in the center of the defensive huddle, who radiated a quiet, calming determination that encouraged his teammates to focus—and Reggie was the moodier young man, apt to exhort teammates to greater heights by being vocal and yelling—then Jackie was the confident loner who stood tall in the back row of the huddle, exuding an almost mystical aura of deep contemplation.

Her stunning good looks are important. No one who knew Jackie disputes that modeling was a realistic option for her. "She was lovely and magnetic," said boys basketball coach Carl Youngstrom. "You couldn't miss her."

Some feel that describing female athletes as "attractive" can be demeaning, but in the age of fit or fat, these same women have ascended to a unique, idealized throne. How does that relate to a sports legacy, though?

Some people possess an indefinable and intangible magnetism, an aura of greatness that exudes from their pores. By all accounts, Jackie Rogers was such a person. Her appearance combined with her talents and demeanor to affect her games and her life on multiple levels. Jackie exuded a charisma that sucked spectators into a tunnel vision, creating an entirely new stature for a high school athlete, male or female, in the 1980s. Only her beauty equaled her joy for the game, and she was way ahead of her time, forming an unparalleled appeal.

Since Don was away at UCLA, Reggie and Loretha had to look out for Jackie, which, given the latter's independence, was no easy task. As willful, powerful people tend to do, Jackie usually did what she wanted. Her Pied Piper nature made people desire to be near her, which, threateningly, included adult men.

Although heady stuff for a 16-year-old girl, Jackie seemed to be developing just fine. She was a minor celebrity, very popular, recognized throughout the city. Even when she wasn't recognized literally, many people felt they'd seen her somewhere. Strangers approached to ask her whether she was a model, whether she'd been on television. *Everyone* wanted to know.

As her brothers before her, though, Jackie was an athlete first— an athlete, oddly enough, who was best known for the sport that may not have been her best.

Don was an All-Northern California basketball player, who played quarterback on the football team. In college he was moved full time to safety, yet later became a first-round NFL draft pick. Reggie was an All-Northern California basketball player, who gave up football when he chose a college, yet later became a first-round NFL draft pick.

True to the breadth of the family's physical gifts, Jackie was a well-known, all-everything basketball player, but her best sport might have been softball. As a pitcher Jackie was alone in the spotlight; but softball, a sport that had almost no fan appeal, was not the place to get attention, so she more likely enjoyed the competition.

What an imposing presence to see the 6-foot-plus Jackie on the mound, her slow, smooth windup obliterated by the blur of her skinny arm slinging the ball past an overmatched hitter at 70 miles per hour.

Before the public cared enough and before newspapers employed enough staff to cover girls' sports with the same intensity as boys', or even to choose all-city teams for softball, the sport existed in anonymity on the small scraggly diamonds at the far end of the campus. One former Norte teacher couldn't remember whether they'd even had a team. No box scores remain. Jackie's true greatness on the diamond remains vivid only in the memories of those who witnessed her feats, who watched her pitch more than a dozen one- or no-hitters.

ONE MOMENT CHANGES EVERYTHING

There's always basketball: a sport where, unlike softball, a long history of records and accomplishment supports Jackie's extreme prowess.

In basketball, as her two brothers had done, Jackie's talent and star quality led Norte to previously unknown heights. After games, bashful competitors would ask for her autograph. But despite what she would accomplish, she would always be the youngest Rogers sibling, and she would always be "just a girl." Don would always be the saint. Reggie had skipped varsity as a sophomore, then missed most of his senior season of football with an injury, gradually developing a reputation as an underachiever who would never be Don. And unlike Don, Jackie was simply too ethereal, beautiful, talented, and too the-third-Rogers-star to be loved by everyone. Days of worship have limited hours—especially around a neighborhood in which so many had so little anyway.

Jackie didn't seem to mind playing second fiddle—not outwardly at least. Not yet. Not as long as she had Don looking out for her, the voice of maturity and reason inside Jackie's cerebral mind. "He was my best friend, and my bodyguard," said Jackie in a recent *Sacramento Bee* interview.

Despite the jealousy welling in Del Paso Heights throughout the early 1980s, when the Rogers are mentioned anywhere in or around Sacramento, most people light up like it's the Fourth of July. In the city's history, before the NBA and the Sacramento Kings arrived and no local colleges played Division I sports, the Rogers were the town's first and preeminent sports celebrities. Because they were three great individual talents and because they came from one family, the Rogers have and had immense staying power.

In 2007—in a more cynical, perhaps more enlightened global world—to imagine three young athletes being worshipped this way is nearly impossible. But the differences between the three Rogers children were already stark, and becoming more so. Had Reggie been 6-foot-even, had he looked like us, had he been more average in size—had he been more like Don—perhaps people would've seen themselves in him, perhaps people would've seen his early struggles as their own. Unfortunately, he wore the curse of the misunderstood giant. When talent is expressed by overwhelming strength or size, Americans tend to root against that package, identifying instead with the underdog. Such is the curse of unparalleled beauty as well. Athletes, especially those of epic size, often seem fantastical, and we imagine how great we would be if we had their God-given advantages, if we were only that tall, that strong. We don't feel as though they even exist in our world, and our social insensitivity to these men proves as much.

Indeed, other types of "greatness" have cynics, as well, and some people felt that Jackie's accomplishments were somehow less substantial because her brothers had come before her. As her athletic achievements attest, though, nothing could have been further from the truth. Americans have such a skewed view of stardom that many believe, as with wealth, stardom would solve all of their problems. Little do they understand that stardom, and the responsibility of stardom, are problems in and of themselves.

Jackie's brothers were stars, yet she also had to contend with the fact that her own mother had been a high school basketball star. How many parents destroy their kids in an attempt to shape them in their own image, determined by impossible standards? No one who lived inside the tiny Olmstead Drive house that the Rogers called home in 1980 was less than six feet tall, or ever achieved anything less than first-team All-City. But Jackie's brothers didn't pitch her games, set her records in points or rebounds, and neither boy led his team to the California State High School basketball championship. As much as Don or Reggie, more so even, Jackie had to find her own way. Even considering Loretha's boundless energy, it still takes a special parent to "get up" emotionally for the 500-plus games of Little League, football, basketball, and track that her mother had to witness before Jackie had played her first high school contest.

Jackie's only advantage on her road to stardom was her ability to practice and play against the very best competition, day in and day out—in her neighborhood and in her own home. Competing against brothers may have helped her hone her talent, but it couldn't have been easy—not with the food issues. The Rogers were that poor, constantly concerned about money. The kids sometimes went to bed hungry; and in a family with the sternly driven Don, the über-talented Reggie, and their feisty mother, pondering the skill necessary to pull a rebound in the family shoot-around or to win the argument over who got to eat the last waffle at breakfast is impossible. A weaker-willed person would've quit sports altogether.

Jackie was Sacramento's biggest female star. No amateur before or since has achieved the fame and notoriety, especially considering the era and the limited exposure and opportunities available to female stars of the time.

Though many boys went to Jackie's games to watch her, astute observers learned how she almost never brought the ball down below her waist, how she almost never dribbled after rebounding the ball beneath the basket. Instead, she would rebound the ball at its highest point, and immediately put it back up in one motion.

A quick perusal of points and rebounds statistics for the Sacramento section in 1982, Reggie's senior year, shows Reggie in the top seven for both points and rebounds. Those stats were gathered from a pool of hundreds of schools in the section, which stretches from the San Francisco Bay area, south to Fresno, and north to the Oregon border. Reggie's performance was great by any measure—one of the best in the state—though it wasn't even the best in his own house. Ever the contented loner, Jackie was also alone statistically. Only a junior, she averaged 19 points and 14 rebounds for Norte Del Rio to rank in the top three in both categories in the section; something neither of her brothers achieved.

Her high game? A 36-point effort—there was no three-point line.

Her high-rebounding total? A 27-board game.

She was named All-City and led Norte Del Rio to the Northern California high school girls' championship game against Los Gatos High School of San Jose.

THE ALL-AMERICA TRAGEDY OF DON ROGERS

Many scouts and reporters were comparing Jackie to Southern California star Cheryl Miller of Riverside Poly High School. A future college Hall of Fame player, and brother of future UCLA and Indiana Pacers star, Reggie, Cheryl Miller's and Jackie's respective games could not have been more different. Jackie had long arms, super-soft hands, a knack for quick put backs. She was not a physical player, but a surprisingly quick-footed ball hawk with a deadly baby hook (no doubt perfected shooting over her brothers). She was always in the right place at the right time, and the ball just seemed to find her. While Jackie may have had height that was comparable to Reggie's, if anything, her instincts for the game more closely resembled Don's.

Cheryl Miller was a new kind of female athlete—perhaps the greatest female athlete of all time, but surely the best at basketball. Cheryl Miller single-handedly began to change the old perception that female athletes lacked explosiveness. Like Jackie, Miller was arguably the best basketball player in a super-talented family. Miller had a complete game and was one of the first women to shoot a true jump shot. A great rebounder—at USC, she led the nation in scoring and rebounding—she was most highly regarded as a slasher who had no difficulty putting the ball on the floor and taking it to the hoop. Driving hard to the basket, then pulling up, tucking her knees, and letting go a tough gliding floater in the lane was the quintessential Miller move—one that no women, and few men, for that matter, could execute as well. Along with the equally impressive McGee sisters—strong, twin towers who dominated inside—Miller brought back-to-back national titles to USC, introducing the women's game to America in the process.

Whether the lithe, airy game of Jackie Rogers would translate to the slogging, physical women's game at the college level remained to be seen. In Jackie Rogers, however, recruiters nationwide saw a future star.

For now, however, as a high school player, Jackie was at the top of her sport and was adding to an already unprecedented family legacy, bringing program-defining wins and underlining them with gaudy personal statistics.

ONE MOMENT CHANGES EVERYTHING

Then, in 1982, just as suddenly and unexpectedly as it began, Norte closed its doors forever.

"It was a combination of things," said Youngstrom, who taught and coached at the school for 25 years, "money, apathy, shrinking enrollment, lack of communication and follow through by the administration. We'd finally broken through athletically, which can sometimes create other opportunities, but the district felt it would be more simple to just shut it down."

The Grant Union District announced that the class of 1982, Reggie's senior year, would be Norte's last, and the student body, including Jackie, and four other returning starters from Norte's section championship team, would be forced to merge with rival Grant, who itself would have four starters returning from one of the top teams in the region.

Even the most optimistic fans of Del Paso Heights girls' sports knew that, while the talent level would be spectacular, blending these bitter rivals into a coherent unit might prove impossible.

Loretha fought the closure tooth and nail. "It was almost over Loretha's dead body," said Larry Brown, principal at Grant High School.

No matter. Something was ending. Don was at UCLA. Reggie was preparing to select a college. And Strawberry Manor, the poorest corner of beguilingly poor Del Paso Heights—the incomparable origin of the Rogers' legacy—was about to lose one of its last rays of sunshine. With the Rogers boys already calling other cities their homes, the closure was like pushing a drowning victim underwater after breathing life back into his lungs.

Norte's closing did have some positives, though—the school would go out on a "high note." No disappointing decline to its depressing past would mark Norte's final days. The school had "broken through" in the minds of Sacramentans, and the idea that Grant and Norte would combine their powerhouse programs sent chills up spines of rival coaches throughout the section. The end also meant that the Rogers would go out on top, that they'd be linked to the school and the school to them forever.

THE ALL-AMERICA TRAGEDY OF DON ROGERS

Some felt that was a fitting tribute, that no second act or comparisons with ensuing generations over the next 100 years could mar their curtain call. Norte would always have the Rogers, who helped make it known. And in many ways, the Rogers would always have Norte.

4

Finally, Sacramento-area talent was beginning to bloom. In 1982, Sacramento's Kevin Wilhite, brother of Broncos running back Gerald Wilhite, was ranked the No. 1 high school back in the country. In basketball, other players besides Reggie stood in line for major scholarships, most notably a pair of rival guards: Ernest Lee from South Sacramento's Kennedy High School, and his Metropolitan League counterpart, Kevin Johnson of Sacramento High. Johnson would go on to star for Cal and later the Phoenix Suns, while Ernest Lee initially would attend the University of Washington.

Reggie was the other big-time Sacramento recruit. One publication listed him as one of the top-16 basketball players in the nation. Despite his Winters-riot injury and his preference for basketball, scouts and coaches from Texas and Oklahoma, to name a couple, still wanted him for football. Some recruited him for both sports, but football seemed the most obvious choice for future stardom. He was fast enough to play tight end, strong enough for the defensive line, but savvy coaches saw him as the new breed of outside linebacker: long-armed and capable of chasing down running backs from sideline to sideline. Even though his grades were merely average, in the more academically liberal 1980s he essentially had his choice of schools.

What continued to befuddle recruiters, though, was Reggie's incessant insistence that football no longer interested him. Moreover, he wasn't interested in the Big Time at all. Despite his top-20 ranking as a basketball player—and that the list of colleges recruiting Reggie were the envy of most players nationwide—he wasn't being courted by Duke, North Carolina, or even UCLA. Football gave him limitless options, and the choice of tradition-rich programs across the country.

Of all his choices—basketball or football, big school or small, where to live, etc.—Reggie shocked everyone early on when he claimed that he wanted to attend the University of Hawaii. The reasons were obvious. He wanted to escape the glare of the mainland (and probably his brother's shadow) and go somewhere far away, a place with no spotlight, absolutely no tradition, and most importantly, no pressure.

"I really loved Hawaii," Reggie said.

In retrospect, it might have been the perfect place for him; but this time, rather than go his own way, Reggie went against his instincts and caved to expectation and pressure. Or perhaps he was finally ready to challenge himself and only needed the opportunity to be presented.

Before their senior years, Reggie and Kennedy High star Ernest Lee met at a California all-star basketball camp in San Diego. The two became fast friends. Lee would become a fixture in the Rogers household. He soon began to date Jackie, and the two fell in love.

Lee was a brash, thickset, 6-foot-3 guard who led the city of Sacramento in scoring and trash talk. He was the area's biggest basketball-only recruit since Bill Cartwright. He had a shaved head and baggy shorts long before they were popular, even before Michael Jordan. And like Jordan, Lee could flat-out sky. Like Don Rogers, he was best known for his rain-bringing jumping ability.

Ernest Lee would scoop up loose balls in traffic and, in one motion, simply go up and hammer down a slam. When inbounding the ball beneath the basket, Kennedy High coach Spider Thomas had designed around a half-dozen plays specifically for Ernest Lee to dunk. One play consisted of a 'wheel' motion where Lee flashed by on the baseline and would receive the ball and reverse jam before continuing right on up the court in one motion—and he never looked back. In the pre-three-point shot era, Lee once had 50 in a single game. While his talent was nationally recognized, though, Ernest did not have the grades of say, a Don Rogers or a Kevin Johnson. In fact, Lee's grades were terrible.

Despite academics-related suspensions and requiring an extra summer to graduate, Ernest still received a unique offer from the University of Washington. Under a special academic-hardship program, he could enroll in school, but he would not be allowed to play or practice with the basketball team for one year, wherein he'd raise his grades to qualifying standards.

Nevada-Las Vegas' Jerry Tarkanian was furious. He accused Washington coach Marv Harshman of stowing Ernest away. Lee couldn't even play for the notorious UNLV Runnin' Rebels, so how had he managed to get into Washington?

Under future Hall of Fame coach Don James, Washington was a football powerhouse. In basketball, longtime coach, Marv Harshman, another future Hall of Fame inductee, led a program that had been consistently good, and had recently challenged UCLA for Pac-10 supremacy. The Huskies were young, played up-tempo, and had a roster dotted with future NBA players, including Germany's Detlef Shrempf. Like the University's athletic department, the city of Seattle was booming. It was beautiful, clean, had numerous progressive business models and a monster music scene. Seattle was fast becoming the hot place to live in America.

As the young men's senior seasons of basketball unfolded, both Reggie and Ernest led their respective teams into the section playoffs, with Norte losing in the first round, but with Lee and Kennedy advancing all the way to the Tournament of Champions in Oakland. Even though his school lost in the middle rounds, they still won enough games and performed well enough to get Lee named to the all-tournament team.

Rogers and Lee were elected first-team All-City by both of Sacramento's newspapers (Reggie made All-Northern California as well). The two friends would end many of their conversations by saying, "See you in the NBA." As a tribute to the stars, both area papers conducted lengthy interviews and ran pictures of the two—good-looking kids with lean physiques, limitless futures, and smiles that stretched from ear to ear—best friends proudly standing side by side.

As the National Letter of Intent deadline approached, Lee had kept after Reggie; and sometime in the spring, Rogers changed his mind about where he wanted to go to school. Lee had managed to convince Reggie to forget about the Islands and come with him to the University of Washington.

Who wouldn't want to have a good friend 600 miles from home? Ernest was Jackie's boyfriend, too. He had a ton of pull with Reggie and obviously influenced him to come to a high-profile Pac-10 institution—one in the same conference as UCLA, where Don Rogers was on the brink of superstardom.

Was basketball truly Reggie's passion, or was he attempting, in his own way, to get out from under Don's shadow? That question emanated from each subsequent decision Reggie would make.

Reggie probably wasn't even certain why he wanted to go to school so far away from his brother. Still, the mutual love and respect that they shared for one another was evident in neighborhood circles. To that point, that positive characteristic belies any mark of a rivalry, friction, or jealousy between the two. Don was like a father to Reggie and Jackie as well as a dutiful son to Loretha. While most older brothers accept the family mantle of leadership and concern, even if just from time to time, all available accounts of Don—from neighbors to teammates to relatives—clearly underline one thing: Don Rogers led his family, and he did so as a matter of course. He accepted and embraced his role from a very early age, and he never once voiced or displayed any amount of weariness whatsoever. Outwardly, leading and caring for others was second nature to Don.

"I have a very nice family," Don told Tracy Dodds of *The Los Angeles Times* in September 1983. "I'm very lucky there."

As for anyone, this was a mixed blessing for Reggie, who on one hand had an absentee father and, on the other, a soft-spoken saint for an older brother. When your natural tendency is to act out rather than conform socially, that concoction can create confusion for a young man about to enter adulthood. Don's standards, though—perhaps the simple threat of his glaring eye—helped keep Reggie in line.

Reggie would soon lose the support of his older brother and face burden of their disparate but enduring legacies. A national tug of war would erupt over which legacy would survive, with Reggie anchoring one end of the rope.

But for now, Reggie only had to endure the saintly Don—the star athlete, the favored son.

5

Unlike the uncertainty surrounding Reggie's college choice, or even his preferred sport, Don and UCLA seemed like a match made in athletic-media heaven—the masterstroke of foresight came courtesy of the Bruins' head coach, Terry Donahue.

Following his highly publicized failure to reestablish the San Francisco 49ers dynasty, and in light of his 2005 dismissal as team president, former UCLA head coach Terry Donahue's once unassailable reputation as a football icon had taken a beating. But with a 49er ownership group uncommitted to winning—forced to play in the worst stadium in the league—and with legend Bill Walsh looking over his shoulder, the opportunity for Donahue to build a winner in San Francisco was never honestly presented. Perhaps Terry Donahue will someday return to the college game, where from 1976-1995 he took UCLA, his alma mater, to 13 bowl games in 20 seasons. Along the way he managed to lead the Bruins to an NCAA-record eight straight postseason wins, including Rose (twice), Fiesta, and Cotton Bowl victories.

Dick Vermeil preceded Donahue at UCLA, but when he left in February 1976 to take over the head coaching duties of the Philadelphia Eagles; Donahue, at age 31, was elevated from offensive coordinator to become the youngest head coach in Pac-10 Conference history. Like most great coaches, especially those who excel at the college game, Donahue had knacks for identifying and developing talent. An innovator who ran a flexible, pro-style offense years before most of the nation caught on, Donahue believed that, to be truly exceptional, his teams needed great safeties anchoring the defense.

With Kenny Easley playing center field in Westwood beginning in 1977, UCLA had the best safety in college football. Not coincidentally, during that same span, the program had begun to achieve consistent success on the field as well. But 1980 was to be Easley's senior season, and Donahue desperately sought a comparably talented replacement to help thwart the potent passing attacks of the Pac-10.

Although many fans around Sacramento shared Donahue's faith in Don Rogers, everyone was still surprised that one of their own would get to be a Bruin. How could he compare to Easley when quaterback, not safety, was his best position? Rogers was obviously a superb athlete, but at that time, in the pre-internet and pre-scouting service era, Sacramento was no football hotbed. Most high schools didn't even film their games. Norte couldn't afford it. UCLA was, to West Coast fans, a sacred golden temple—a glamorous, fantasy destination way down south in the City of Angels. By contrast, before Don, most of the capitol city's football talent had dreams so modest, that the "ultimate" was an invitation to try out at hometown Division II Sacramento State. Terry Donahue saw something in Rogers, though. Not a man prone to praise, when the UCLA coach proclaimed—to Los Angeles' dubious football fans—that this kid from the Central Valley could be the next great UCLA safety their eyes rolled faster than a 7.0 San Andreas temblor.

A three-time, first-team consensus All-American (1978-1980), many journalists consider Easley the greatest safety in college football history. To make their argument even more compelling, they didn't have to travel far to find No. 2. Southern Cal's Ronnie Lott, like Easley, would become a charter member of the Top-100 all-time college football players club. A 2002 inductee to the College Football Hall of Fame, Lott was knocking receivers unconscious at the Coliseum while Kenny Easley was sending them to the trainer's room with incurable cases of "the drops."

THE ALL-AMERICA TRAGEDY OF DON ROGERS

Needless to say, West Coast football fans had a solid indication of what great safeties looked like.

But so did Terry Donahue.

Many fans regarded his predictions as proof that he'd lost his mind—he'd OD'd on sunshine. They, justifiably, considered it nothing more than elevated hype. Sacramento was nowhere-ville to Pacific Ocean sophisticates, and their self-proclaimed oracular abilities led them to believe that, with Easley and Lott set to graduate in the spring of 1981, a precipitous decline in talent awaited defensive backfields of both local college powers.

They were dead wrong.

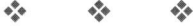

In his recruitment of Don, Donahue didn't mince words or actions. With hard work, Rogers could be a star—and on a Kenny Easley level. But Easley was an once-in-a-lifetime player, so why put that kind of pressure on an unknown?

Those who understood Donahue, and those journalists who covered UCLA, also knew that the coach was a no-nonsense mentor and motivator. With his thick hair and perfect tan, he may have looked like a handsome surfer, or at least a former quarterback, but he was neither. UCLA's head coach had played defensive tackle in college. He was not a typical, clichéd Left Coaster playing fast-break football and creating zany, tricky offensive schemes. Donahue liked players who could clean clocks, and the players on his Bruin defenses were experts at stopping time.

Backing up his gutsy predictions, Donahue tied Don and Easley together at the hip, assigning the freshman to room with All-Everything Easley on the road from the moment he set foot on the Westwood campus. He also stuck Rogers in locker stall No. 7, a cubicle away from Easley's now retired No. 5 spot.

The effect on Don living with and being mentored by the great Kenny Easley was pronounced and lasting. "From the moment I arrived in Westwood, Kenny took me under his wing," said Rogers before his senior season. "I came to UCLA because of Kenny. I owe everything I am as a football player to him."

Littered with ability and blessed with arriving talent, UCLA's football team boasted several future notables, including quarterback Tom Ramsey, flanker Karl Dorrell—a pre-med major and future UCLA head football coach—monstrous tackles Irv Eatman and Luis Sharpe, and running back Freeman McNeil. Quarterbacks Rick Neuheisel, who would become a successful college coach at Colorado and Washington, and Steve Bono, who as backup to Joe Montana and Steve Young with the 49ers was known as the best and highest-paid third-string player in NFL history, wore Bruin blue alongside Don as well.

Don spent his freshman season in 1980 observing road-roommate Easley accumulate tackles, interceptions, and awards. "I watched his every move," said Don.

The Bruins finished 9-2, including a non-conference sweep of the Big Ten's Purdue, Wisconsin, and Ohio State, allowing only 14 points total in the three games. A huge reason for the defense's success was that, because of Easley, teams couldn't—or wouldn't—throw deep against the Bruins, who were then able to stack the line against the run. Never mind throwing down the middle, if the receiver even dared to catch the ball, Easley would make him pay.

After his senior season, for the third straight year, Easley earned consensus first team All-America honors, and was voted All-Pac 10 first team for a record fourth year. He finished ninth in the Heisman Trophy balloting, and established UCLA career records of 324 tackles and 19 interceptions.

With Easley taking almost every meaningful snap that season, backup Rogers played mostly on special teams, recording five unassisted tackles—hardly an indicator of what was to come—but his teammates saw the potential.

"Don came in strong, and got better every day," said a former UCLA teammate, a sentiment widespread enough to earn Don the team's Most Improved Player award at season's end.

Don was in no way a one-dimensional player, though—he was also serious about his studies. He majored in economics; and, knowing how how much he had sacrificed to become the first in his family to attend college, he wasn't about to take any chances. The value of a UCLA degree in the real world did not escape him; nor did the importance of setting a good example for Reggie and Jackie. Others, such as Terry Donahue, predicted greatness for him on the gridiron, but nothing distracted Don, who maintained a 3.0 grade-point average throughout his college career.

"He was a model player and citizen," said a former coach, who then added, rather ominously: "In fact, it seemed like he refused to goof off at all."

Players such as Kenny Easley aren't simply born on a Tuesday afternoon. They go a long way toward creating themselves through hard work and discipline; and Easley knew well the toil that went into preparing for games off the field. He stressed to Don the importance of practicing hard, taking care of his body, and studying game films of opponents. "Prepare yourself for each game every way you can," Easley told Rogers. "You play the way you practice, so you've got to practice hard."

Personal accountability is the first great hurdle athletes must clear when they graduate from high school sports to Division I. Talent can allow a star to be a star for a while, but everyone hits a wall unless they learn to prepare, work hard, and do the little things to keep their skills attuned. At the highest levels of sport, *everyone* is talented. Few of Easley's lessons were lost on Don, who desperately wanted to achieve all the great things his mentor had accomplished. Neither player partied or drank much. They worked out like demons on earth's final day, becoming kindred spirits who vowed to remain close for life.

His freshman season complete, Don had to say goodbye to someone who would forever hold a special place in his life. Teammates, roommates, UCLA Bruins, safeties, consummate athletes, mentor and pupil, Easley had taught Don more than Terry Donahue could have hoped, or imagined. In six short months, Don had learned what it meant to be a football player—and a man.

In the April 1981 NFL Draft, the Seattle Seahawks selected Easley with the fourth overall pick. Despite having played no college basketball, so much was thought of his athleticism, leadership, ball-hawking skills, and approach to athletics, the NBA's Chicago Bulls drafted Easley as well.

Once in the NFL Easley picked up right where he'd left off at UCLA. After recording three interceptions and a touchdown in his first season, Easley was named the 1981 AFC Defensive Rookie of the Year. Starting in his second season, he was named All-Pro five straight times. In 1983, he was named AFC Defensive Player of the Year; and in 1984, after snatching ten interceptions, he claimed that award once again. The Seahawks franchise rewarded him by making the much-loved Easley the highest-paid defensive player in the league. In a recent survey of Seattle sports fans, along with Hall of Fame wide receiver and Oklahoma congressman Steve Largent, Easley was voted one of the five most popular athletes in the Emerald City's history. In 2002, at halftime of a game against the San Francisco 49ers, Kenny Easley was inducted into the Seattle Seahawks Ring of Honor.

All too often, professional careers overshadow college achievement. Injuries, poor decisions, ill-fitting coaching philosophies, and just plain bad luck create the many monsters that can devour a player's NFL success and even reach back to undermine his college reputation. What hinders Easley's argument as the greatest safety ever would also hamper the reputation of his close friend, and protégé, Don Rogers.

Easley's professional career ended mysteriously, and many fans aren't sure why.

In 1988, after seven years in the NFL, Easley began to wonder whether he was feeling the toll that years of violent collisions had taken on his body—or so he thought. A nagging ankle injury that had caused him to miss part of the 1986 season would come back to haunt him in 1988, and well beyond.

In a startling irony, to dull the pain of Easley's throbbing ankle, Seahawk physicians gave him over-the-counter Advil. For months, he took the pills without so much as a second thought. Two years later, prior to the 1988 season, Easley was undergoing a standard physical examination when a blood test revealed damage to his

THE ALL-AMERICA TRAGEDY OF DON ROGERS

kidneys—damage so severe that an ambulance was summoned immediately.

Prolonged use of Advil was believed to be the cause. After lawsuits and much acrimony, the gentlemanly, soft-spoken Easley was estranged from the Seahawks, which made them reluctant to promote his legacy and accomplishments following his retirement, further hindering the staying power of his reputation. More importantly, however, Easley's damaged kidney put his life in danger, and within two years, he would need a transplant.

After a sterling seven-year NFL career that saw the accumulation of every possible honor, as well as the theft of 32 interceptions, Kenny Easley's career ended suddenly before the 1988 season began.

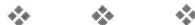

In 1981, Southern California had a void to fill.

Two of the first eight picks of the spring NFL draft had been used to select Pac-10 safeties from Los Angeles, Kenny Easley and Ronnie Lott, both once-in-a-generation-type players. Before Easley and Lott, rarely had one safety—and never had two—been selected in the first eight picks. Left tackles, running backs, quarterbacks, middle linebackers, and defensive ends had always been positional draft priorities.

Traditionally, safeties were cerebral centerfielders who may lack the athleticism of cornerbacks, the hands of receivers, or the size of linebackers, but compensate for any physical shortcomings with brains, preparation, and tenacity.

With his mentor, Easley, and his mentor's friendly rival, Ronnie Lott, off to the NFL, much of the city's football focus was on Don. The standard to bear was unmatched in college football history. Everyone wanted to know: Could Don Rogers really maintain the level of excellence establish by those who preceded him?

In a word: Absolutely.

"When I was 12," said longtime NFL safety Marcus Robertson on a fan website in 2002, "I had a poster of Easley and a poster of

ONE MOMENT CHANGES EVERYTHING

Don Rogers on my bedroom door. Along with Ronnie Lott, they brought respect to the position; and from then on, I wanted to be a safety."

Over at USC, the Trojans had All-America safeties throughout the 1980s. Dennis Smith was there in 1980, then Lott in 1980 and '81, and later Tim McDonald and Mark Carrier—all Pro Bowl-caliber NFL players. In terms of safety talent, however, UCLA played second fiddle to no team. With Kenny Easley and Don Rogers, the Bruins had built their own pipeline of All-America and star NFL safeties.

In 1981, Don's UCLA career finally began in earnest. His highly anticipated sophomore debut came in the Bruins' 31-13 romp over Big Ten school Wisconsin: Rogers led the team with 11 unassisted tackles and recorded his first career interception. He was everywhere—blanketing receivers, batting passes, chasing down sweeps, stuffing the gaps to suffocate the Badger running game. He didn't play a perfect game, but he was an immediate fan favorite. By the second half, rather than risk further collisions with the 6-foot-1, 208-pound Rogers, the Badger receivers were pulling up lame and dropping passes left and right.

Experienced college football fans can see when a player has risen above his competition. Fans of UCLA knew right away that Don was something special, something that went beyond statistical success. Don appeared to be playing at a higher rate of speed than other players, at a different intensity level. As a former sprinter, all that was possible for Don, but the difference between football speed and track speed is vast; and that distinction lies in the player's instincts and angles of pursuit. Don was simply faster to the ball. His explosiveness allowed him to leap for the ball—or a hit—at the highest point.

Don was intensely physical—even more so than Easley. When Don collided with a ball carrier, squeamish spectators averted their eyes, startled by the loud, painful *pop* that brought them all too close to the violent impact.

The Wisconsin game was a clear indicator of things to come. Only a sophomore, Don would lead the 1981 Bruins in tackles with 133—more than UCLA record holder and good friend Kenny Easley had ever recorded in a single season. He caused half a dozen fumbles, picked off three passes, and knocked down a dozen more. He made All-Pac 10 Conference, but more importantly, he showed Los Angeles that the city's emerging legacy of star safeties would carry on seamlessly.

The Bruins finished the 1981 season with a respectable 7-4-1 record that culminated with a 33-14 loss to Michigan—a team they would play twice the following year—in the now-defunct Astro Bluebonnet Bowl, held in the Astrodome in Houston, Texas.

Back in Sacramento, as his brother had done, senior Reggie Rogers was named to the All-Northern California basketball team. Enduring double and triple teams, Reggie still managed to average 22 points and 14 rebounds per game, leading Norte to a 23-5 overall record and a spot in the sectional playoffs, where they lost a hard-fought game in the first round to Sacramento-city power Cordova.

With nearly identical stats as Reggie, Jackie, just a junior, led Norte through the sectional playoffs and into the Tournament of Champions at the Oakland Coliseum Arena against the other sectional champions from Northern and Central California. Winning four games, the Norte girls breezed their way to the Final Four where, despite Jackie's 18 second-half points, they lost to Los Gatos High School of San Jose, falling just one win short of facing the Southern California champion in the state final.

Then, Norte Del Rio High School shut its doors forever in June 1982.

While both her brothers would be away at college, Jackie and her Norte basketball teammates would have to finish high school across the neighborhood at rival Grant. Grant's girls certainly didn't want Norte's players stealing their thunder. As they would for the next ten consecutive seasons, Grant's varsity girls had qualified for the section playoffs again during the 1981-82 year, and would be returning most of the squad the following season.

Just how much effort the district's administrators put into finding a way to mesh two powerhouse basketball programs

ONE MOMENT CHANGES EVERYTHING

became evident when they announced that Norte's longtime boys head basketball coach, Carl Youngstrom, would assist Grant's highly regarded Steve Williams. For the classy Youngstrom, who—even with a white-hot reputation thanks to the Rogers Bros.—was nearing retirement, the "demotion" was offset by his respect for Williams. The combined student bodies guaranteed that Grant, a traditional area sports power, would have a clamp on Del Paso Heights talent.

The transition for the girls was not nearly so simple. It wasn't just a matter of putting Jackie in the middle and surrounding her with Grant players. She may have been Norte's glamorous star, but the school had been blessed with two other six-footers as well, one of whom, like Jackie, was considered a serious Division I prospect. A power play for the girls' head-coaching basketball job at Grant soon followed; and, in a highly publicized move that reeked of bureaucratic good intention, one that still causes resentment today, the district administrators replaced Grant's longtime head coach with Norte's less experienced leader, Don Boyce.

Norte's girls' team had only been a power since Jackie's enrollment, but with her leading the way they were one of the final four teams in California in 1982. Not a bad breakthrough season. As for Grant's girls—although not yet a state final four school—they had won 20 games, qualifying them for the sectional playoffs. In girls' sports, as well as in boys, Grant was one of the preeminent Sacramento Valley powers in athletics, but especially in basketball. The school's girls' squad had reached the Tournament of Champions in Oakland more times than any other school in section history. But awkward coaching changes in sports are what happen when non-sports people—bureaucrats—make well-intentioned, but ultimately naïve decisions regarding personnel in an arena where success is measured by victories and nothing less.

It is, however, only high school, and ideally, sports should not be the priority. That is, unless you live in a lower-income neighborhood where a majority of the student body comes from single-parent homes unable to afford college, where a sports scholarship is a golden ticket. The chosen successor to the head coaching position for a longtime power program would definitely matter more in this case, exponentially more than it would elsewhere.

The returning Grant players' anxieties over the new Norte girls, as well as the coaching change, is best described by a former Grant player. "We didn't want them (Norte's girls) here. We didn't know what to expect. We hung out with our team, and they sort of stayed with their teammates."

In the end, however, it didn't matter. The Grant High School Pacers, flush with the talented towers Jackie and 6-foot Tori Hunt, as well as several other former Dons players, would begin the 1982-1983 season ranked No. 1 in the Sacramento Section, top five in Northern California.

Yet, even that lofty ranking would soon prove to be far too low.

6

Alongside Ernest Lee, Reggie had begun freshman classes at the University of Washington, making him not only the second member of his family to attend college, but the second sibling to earn a Pac-10 scholarship as well. Loaded with talent, the Huskies hoops team was led by head coach Marv Harshman, who felt that, in Reggie, he had found the bruising inside player he needed to deflect pressure off his elegant shooting guard, Paul Fortier, and his smooth, 6-foot-9 German swingman, Detlef Shrempf. The latter, due to his dexterity, was becoming known as "the white Magic Johnson" in various basketball circles.

Adjusting to college life was as difficult for Reggie as it is for many teenagers, but he had a secret weapon—Don—and many evenings, the two would talk by phone late into the night. Still, Reggie never really had been more than a few miles from home. And, if Reggie was having typical freshman adjustment issues, roommate and friend Ernest Lee was already in big trouble.

"There was a lot of confusion about money," Reggie told the *Sacramento Bee*.

For Reggie, who was on scholarship, money wasn't a real problem. Ernest, however, a probationary admit, had little guidance and no money. Coming from the same background as Reggie, a poor, broken home (Lee had not had contact with his father in years), Ernest had to struggle just to get enough to eat. Though some would say that, as unprepared as Ernest was for the rigors of college—that he never really had a chance—he soon made a decision that would have dire consequences for both young men.

ONE MOMENT CHANGES EVERYTHING

After only a few months on campus, Ernest dropped out of school; and for a while, at least, the pair's mantra changed from "See you in the NBA" to "Whatever happened to Ernest Lee?" Ernest Lee all but vanished from the public eye. Yet, he would soon reappear in spectacular fashion to claim the basketball legacy he had always imagined.

Down in Los Angeles, Don was beginning his junior year at UCLA. For his third season in Westwood, the Bruins were returning almost everyone from the previous year's 7-4-1 squad. The national media had noticed, and the Associated Press had UCLA ranked in the Top 20 to begin the season.

Jackie was at talent-rich Grant, and every school in the country was recruiting her for basketball. So with Reggie at nationally ranked Washington and Don leading his Bruins into another season of high expectations, the entire Rogers Clan had opened its golden era of greatness—a time when they could do no wrong, when the future was limitless, and when journalists, swept up in the certainty of a happy ending, wrote blazing accounts of the family's rags-to-coming-riches saga.

Everyone was happy—and it seemed that everyone would remain happy, so long as Don Rogers was leading the way.

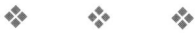

Momentum is the most misunderstood phenomenon in life, and sports are no different. Scientists, professors, and fortune tellers talk about how "luck" affects individuals, games, teams, families, seasons, programs, and even generations. And true, for lack of a better definition, the way the ball bounces, and who it bounces to, can be seen as luck. But luck is not personal and has no preference. A person may make some of their own, but for the most part, luck comes and goes to all people equally. But momentum, which is intangible and often goes dismissed as "mere luck," is different. For individuals, personal momentum is bigger than mere chance. It churns inside us, connecting us to our families via blood, events, and decisions that occurred generations before we were born.

THE ALL-AMERICA TRAGEDY OF DON ROGERS

Good or bad, luck doesn't last. No statistics exist to prove this, but most people will have the exact same amount of good in their lives as bad. While driving a car, a person will hit just as many green lights as red ones. Everyone. But having momentum is different. Teams can win ten championships in a row. A financial investor can make the right call almost every single time. Momentum is something beyond luck, but isn't the mere result of hard work. Momentum can be inside you or, as with a team or family, inside something of which you are a part. It begins with your ancestors, or is found in the history of a particular university's sports teams from decades before you were born. Momentum can be good or bad—it is genetic, it's social, and it's everywhere and nowhere, all at once. Momentum is "luck" on steroids, or it's luck with hard work and expectation and habit—as in getting in the habit of winning or succeeding. Or losing. And for good or ill, that takes time to ingrain.

One other component bears examination: Momentum is easier lost than found.

For the Rogers siblings, the 1982-83 academic year opened doors to the national coming-out party for one of the all-time greatest familial eras in sports history. The Rogers had the all-important momentum behind them. Don ignited an upward thrust that was now fueled by athletics, which served as the boosters for the rocket that was lifting the family beyond the dense atmosphere of failure surrounding Del Paso Heights and their own family's history. No longer were they subject to the typical Strawberry Heights destiny. No longer would they have to succumb.

And it all began with Don, who seemed to take the responsibility of leading his family out and up in stride.

However, with Reggie, Jackie and Loretha, 19-year-old Don Rogers now had someone else to consider. Over the previous summer, Don had briefly dated a girl who was a cheerleader at Grant; and sometime during his sophomore season, Don learned that he was going to be a father. Today, more babies are born out of wedlock in America than to married couples; but in 1982, the percentage was far lower, and many people considered it a cultural tragedy. At such a young age, a child seemed like a one-way ticket to a life of hardship.

Only a teenager, Don still had made, until then, all the right decisions concerning his life. While this might appear to be the first chink in Don's otherwise-pristine armor—something that could force him to drop out of school, quit football, and find a job—having made the sacrifices to achieve the grades he needed to get into UCLA and to keep himself in top shape, Don approached this situation no differently. He announced to his mother and the girl's family that he was determined to be more than an adequate dad, and promised to be an exceptional father. Collectively, they all decided that Don should continue at UCLA, and Loretha volunteered to take an active role in raising the child. Although Don and the child's mother never considered marriage, they maintained a strong friendship, which would pay off immeasurably in the not-too-distant future.

It's impossible to know exactly what Don was thinking at the time. He was just a kid, and fatherhood could not have come as good news to someone with his eye on the NFL. Yet, as the Rogers' legacy unfolds, the baby, who they named Don Jr.—whom everyone would call "Little D"—would become one of the best things to happen to the enigmatic family.

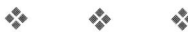

A son at home in Sacramento, a brother in Seattle, and sister at Grant High School—it was time for the Rogers family to take the next step toward their own futures.

"Donny had a good year for us last year and with the experience he gained," UCLA coach Terry Donahue told *The Los Angeles Times* in the summer of 1982. "He's going to be an even better player this year. He stepped into the position vacated by the best defensive back we've ever had here (Easley), and handled it with maturity."

THE ALL-AMERICA TRAGEDY OF DON ROGERS

The 1982 UCLA football season would be one of the best in school history. Don assumed the leader's role on defense, and watching him play left much of his competition feeling a slight twinge of embarrassment. He devastated ball carriers with his hitting, using his blazing speed and rock-solid physique to dominate games in a manner that few safeties had ever done.

In a perfect world, those of us who could never play like Don Rogers would be quelled by his unlikable nature, his idiocy, his bravado. The world isn't perfect, though, and an *unlikable* Don Rogers didn't seem to exist. Quiet, composed, just, exhorting his teammates to greater heights—both on and off the field, Don was the most popular Bruin on campus in *any* sport. His opponents singled him out as one of the greatest football players of his, or any, generation.

After UCLA beat Michigan 31-27 early in the 1982 season, a game in which the Wolverines once led by 21 points, Michigan All-America wide receiver Anthony Carter and Don sang one another's praises. Regarding an infamous hit Don laid on Carter in the Bruins' come-from-behind victory in Ann Arbor, Rogers said, "I saw that Smith (Michigan's quarterback) was going to go to him (Carter), so I ran up and got a good, solid shot on him, right in the chest. I really hit him hard." Rogers, who had 15 tackles in the game, at first, didn't think that Carter would be able to get up.

When it became apparent that A.C. was going to be okay, Don said to him, "That was a pretty good hit, wasn't it?" Carter, the fourth-place Heisman finalist that year, jumped up and replied, "I got the first down, didn't I?"

After the game, Rogers went on to say, "Carter's amazing for a little guy. He can really take a hit on top of being so quick and having such great hands."

Before the two teams met later that season in the Rose Bowl, Carter would say, "That was the one time (Rogers' hit) I got hurt bad enough that I wondered to myself, 'What are you doing out here?' I think it shocked him when I got up."

Throughout the 1982 season opponents always had to know where No. 7 was; and combined with shutdown cornerback Lupe

ONE MOMENT CHANGES EVERYTHING

Sanchez, UCLA's pass defense did indeed control a good portion of the field, which required teams to alter their game plans to stay away from the duo as much as possible. The Bruins' 10 wins in 1982 were the most by UCLA in almost 40 years and culminated in a 24-14 win over Michigan in the January 1, 1983, Rose Bowl. On one of the biggest stages in sports, in front of 103,000 fans and a worldwide television audience, Anthony Carter endured one of his worst days as a collegian with five catches for a pedestrian 59 yards.

Though the game's outcome was never really in doubt, the contest was overshadowed by one of the greatest hits in college football history. Creative journalists struggled to find the words to describe Rogers' second-quarter collision with Michigan quarterback Steve Smith; and in the end, old standbys best captured the moment.

"Bone-jarring," said the UCLA media guide.

"Game-changing," recalled *The Sacramento Union.*

"Smashing," and "jolting," claimed *The Los Angeles Times.*

Twenty years later, Terry Donahue would say, "Don turned the Rose Bowl around with one of the greatest hits I've ever seen—knocked their quarterback out of the game with one of those plays you never forget."

Michigan quarterback Steve Smith faked a pitch on an option play and turned upfield. He was met in the gap by Don, who had 20 yards of open field to utilize his 9.8-second 100-yard dash speed to pick up momentum. Smith suffered a separated shoulder on the play, and, like Michigan, was through for the day.

On January 2, the morning after the game, *The Los Angeles Times* published a nearly full-page color photo (as did dozens of newspapers around the country) in which Don is little more than a threatening blur as Smith braces for impact. Beneath the photo is a large caption that reads, "Mr. Rogers' Neighborhood." And beneath that, a smaller caption reads, "It wasn't a Friendly Place for Some Tourists From Michigan."

The article begins, "Steve Smith, Michigan's starting quarterback, will remember Don Rogers—and may grimace with

THE ALL-AMERICA TRAGEDY OF DON ROGERS

pain at the thought—for some time." The inevitable Kenny Easley comparisons arrive next, as the journalist begins to compare facial similarities of Rogers and his mentor. Typical to his credo, Don credits Easley with his own progress as a player, but tells the reporter that he "doesn't try to copy Easley's style, only that he (Easley) instilled in him the incentive to be a tough defender."

Elected the game's MVP, Don became the first defensive player in the bowl's nearly 80-year history to win the award. His hit on Smith, as well as UCLA's second victory of the season over Michigan, began to change the perception that the "surfer boys" in the sky-blue jerseys from L.A. were soft. Yet, it had an impact on people other than Smith. High school and Pop Warner players who favored the defensive side of the ball had a new hero. Receivers around the country tried to convince themselves that the glory of touchdowns was worth the pain and suffering that safeties built like Sherman tanks could engender.

Realizing that Don was just a junior, wide receivers at colleges all across the nation checked their team's schedules to see if UCLA and Don were on the slate for 1983. UCLA finished 1982 ranked No. 5 in the nation, but with the sweep of Michigan, another blowout of Wisconsin, a romp over Colorado, and their 5-1-1 Pac-10 record (their lone loss was by three-points at No. 6 Washington), many felt that UCLA's final No. 5 national ranking was too low. One thing that was not 'too low' was Don's reputation. He had once again led the Bruins in tackles with 124 stops, including an astounding 94 solo takedowns. He intercepted four passes, and in an often-violent fashion, he broke up 15 more. After the season, Don was named first-team All-Pac 10, and honorable mention All-America.

Yet, as Don compiled big games and accolades, 400 miles north of UCLA and the Rose Bowl, up Interstate 5 in Sacramento, Jackie Rogers and the Grant High School Pacers had managed to meet everyone's highest expectations as well.

ONE MOMENT CHANGES EVERYTHING

❖ ❖ ❖

Players on every blacktop in America—in every city, in every state—think the toughest ball played goes down right where they stand. But make no mistake: California takes a backseat to no region when it comes to producing competitors, professional athletes, even Olympians. When a team sets records in the Golden State, they do so against the best talent in the country.

The 1983 Grant Pacers dominated everything in their path. The petty friction that threatened to emerge when Norte closed was dispelled as the magic of their potential greatness took hold. Of approximately 1,000 high schools, Grant had risen to an unprecedented No. 2 ranking in the state—the best ever for a team from the Capitol. On their way to still-standing California state records of most overall wins in a single season and most consecutive wins in a single season (36), they'd breezed through their league, their section, and the TOC in Oakland.

Grant was preparing for the state final, where they would face Southern California's Ventura Buena High School. The *Sacramento Bee* ran a detailed preview of the Grant Pacers on the front page the morning of the game, as well as an article outlining what the Pacers would have to do to go undefeated. The consensus was that, to win the state title, Jackie would have to lead the way.

The Ventura Buena High School program was in the middle of a ten-year run that would see them emerge victorious an incomprehensible 94 percent of the time (246-16). And the 1983 VBHS team may well have been the best ever. Yet, with Jackie, fellow six-footer Tori Hunt, who was a more physical player, and an outstanding holdover trio of guards, the Pacers had entered the sectional playoffs with a 26-0 record and a No. 5 state ranking. Jackie's scoring and rebounding averages suffered due to their many blowouts, but she easily maintained a place among the sectional top ten in both categories. She also made first-team All-City, All-Section, and was runner-up for MVP at the TOC in Oakland.

Still, something was different for her. At times, she seemed listless and lacked enthusiasm. Her effervescence seemed flat, and others noticed. And when Grant lost the 1983 state championship to Venture Buena—who would again win the state title the following year in 1984—people began to wonder whether her brothers' collective absence had affected her motivation.

After contributing to a never-before-seen 36-1 record, Jackie had to pick a college. Without a major university to call its own, Sacramento has always been a Pac-10 town; and from a list of 50 schools, she became the record third child from one family to accept a scholarship to a Pac-10 university. On the surface, Jackie's decision seemed reasonable: Under head coach Aki Hill, Oregon State was a perennial 20-game winner and postseason qualifier. Her choice didn't produce regional ripples or curious whispers, but some closer to her were vexed. Why had this urbane young woman, who seemed to like the bright lights and could go wherever she wanted, select a school in the tiny town of Corvallis, Oregon?

Perhaps it was just a coincidence that Don became Rose Bowl MVP only a few weeks before Jackie led Grant to the state finals. But on the same day that the Sacramento Sectional girls' playoffs began, Reggie Rogers' first ever Pac-10 league game as a Washington Husky took place at UCLA's Pauley Pavilion in Westwood. Don brought out almost the entire Rose Bowl champion football team to watch his brother perform—and as the game wore on, the Bruins surely ribbed him about letting his brother commit to their northern rivals.

Truth was, UCLA hadn't recruited Reggie for basketball, but by the end of the day, he made them wish they had. He exacted his revenge on the Bruins with a spectacular afternoon. Reggie, who stood only 6-foot-6, lined up at center, where he led all scorers with 22 points and a dozen rebounds as the Huskies notched an easy 30-point victory.

Thus, farther down that same front page of the *Sacramento Bee* featuring the preview on Jackie, the paper ran an Associated Press article with the following headline:

"Freshman Leads Washington to Victory Over UCLA"

ONE MOMENT CHANGES EVERYTHING

The 1982–1983 Huskies would finish .500, and Reggie made the All-Pac 10 freshman team. As soon as the season concluded, he received a letter telling him that he was being considered as a potential member of the 1984 United States Olympic basketball team—in Los Angeles.

Early '80s Sacramento had no professional sports teams, no college teams, and at that time, finding a city of comparable size—a state capitol with two daily newspapers—with less to offer its citizenry would have been nearly impossible. But imagine the star power of the Rogers kids in the pre-cable era. Their multisport dominance, the overall appeal of native children shining beneath bright lights in Seattle and Los Angeles, spawned hundreds of articles each year. This was not 2007, the era of single-sport high school specialists and press conferences to announce college choices nationwide each day.

Three kids now carried the weight of an entire city on their shoulders. The question was, "How would they respond?"

7

The 1983 UCLA football media guide has a cover photo of Don: Eyes locked in on a target, pronounced forward lean to his sprint, wrists tightly wrapped in white tape, Don looks to make a hit, and the Bruins are preparing to build on the previous season's 10-1-1 record. Below, the caption reads: "Rose Bowl Champions." By now, everyone knew who Don was. Being MVP of the Rose Bowl has that effect on football fans. Knocking the opponents' quarterback out of the game with a perfectly delivered hit hadn't hurt Rogers' name recognition, either.

Even though the sudden fame and notoriety were difficult for the down-to-earth Don Rogers to digest, he was selected for the *Playboy* preseason All-America team. He was then flown down to the Florida *Playboy* mansion, where he was photographed with the likes of fellow *Playboy* All-Americans Irving Fryar and Mike Rozier of Nebraska, linebacker Jack Del Rio of rival USC, defensive back Terry Hoage from Georgia, and linebacker Wilber Marshall of Florida. Don called the experience one of the best of his life. To be recognized before his senior season—to be named to what was, at the time, the most prestigious All-America team in the country—gave Don the sense that he truly had arrived.

If all the glamour and glory were going to Don's head, though, no one noticed. He doubled his efforts to make sure his family knew he was there, and his teammates say that he called someone in his family every day, also speaking with Little D's mother regularly. While Reggie, Jackie, and Loretha all wanted to hear

ONE MOMENT CHANGES EVERYTHING

about Don's experiences, he typically deflected attention away from himself, focusing the conversation on them instead.

Don's reputation soared, and he neared the superstar levels of Ronnie Lott and his mentor, Kenny Easley. Keeping with tradition, Terry Donahue even asked Don to room with UCLA freshman safety James Washington on the road. Don was the unquestioned leader of the Bruins.

In 1983, however, the youthful UCLA team had few experienced players back from the '82 squad that finished 10-1-1. To make matters even more difficult, No. 1 Nebraska, No. 5 Georgia, and No. 7 Brigham Young awaited on the non-conference schedule. Added to three games against ranked teams from the Pac-10, the Bruins gauntlet was the toughest nationwide. Four teams they would face had won, would win, or would share a national title within a three-year span.

Before the season, Georgia's Herschel Walker had done the unthinkable and had left school a year early to join the fledgling USFL. Walker had been terrorizing college players for three years, and the thought was that the Bulldogs might not be as good without their star tailback. The opposite was true, however, as UCLA's season began with a 19-8 loss to Georgia at Sanford Stadium in Athens, which was followed by a 26-26 tie with Arizona State then a humiliating 42-10 loss to a Nebraska team that many consider to be one of the most talented college football teams of all time. The following week, the Bruins fell again, 35-37 to 1984 national champion BYU.

Then something clicked in Westwood. UCLA started making plays and winning the close games that they couldn't finish off earlier in the year, recording five straight wins before losing a nail biter to Arizona. Yet, after finishing the regular season with a 27-17 victory over rival USC, the Bruins' 6-1-1 conference record still meant another Pac-10 title and another trip to the Rose Bowl, where they would be a nearly 20-point underdog to 10-1 Big Ten Champion, Illinois.

As any coach will say, though, it's what happens off the field that affects outcomes. On his Christmas holiday, Don had the chance to visit his family in Sacramento. As he usually did, he stopped by the Robertson Community Center, which was a magnet for kids and a safe gathering place for athletes from all over Del Paso Heights. Don was shooting baskets, running up and down the court without breaking a sweat, as he spotted Gayland Houston entering the gym.

Houston had been Grant High School's star running back, and a national football prospect that had just returned from a recruiting trip to the University of Illinois, the Bruins' upcoming Rose Bowl opponent. Don, who was a hero to every kid in The Heights—especially the athletes—went over to chat with Houston.

If what Houston told Don shocked him, Rogers didn't show it.

It seemed that on his recruiting trip the previous weekend in Champaign, Illinois, the Illini players had told Houston that, not only were they were going to destroy UCLA in the Rose Bowl, but that Don Rogers was overrated, and that Pac-10 football was soft. "I'm from California, and they don't play serious football like we do in the Big Ten," a tall, lanky wide receiver had told Houston.

Witnesses verify that Don listened intently, his kind, accepting grin never leaving his face, before assuring Houston in his trademark soft voice, that Illinois was indeed "a very good school and a great team." He then told Houston that he should go to school wherever he felt the most comfortable.

All around the recreation center, probably unbeknownst to Don, the buzz of games and the noise of kids playing had stopped. Del Paso Heights is a Mecca of single-parent households, most of which lack a father figure. Everyone was quietly listening to Don counsel Houston, inching ever closer in the hope that he too would someday merit a conference. Those who knew Don, the "regulars" at the Robertson Community Center, understood that he was nothing if not approachable. Don never turned down a reasonable request, just so long as the person making that request asking promised that he or she did their homework as their teachers told them. Like a politician kissing a baby, it's often lip service when an athlete tells a young kid to "Stay in school and study." To Don Rogers, however, getting an education was serious business, and the kids around the neighborhood all knew it.

This day, Don wanted to make sure that Houston knew that the Pac-10 was one of the best conferences in the country, and that the universities in the league had much to offer. Before leaving, he told Houston that school was an important decision, and that he should watch the Rose Bowl before deciding which conference was stronger.

In the most one-sided Rose Bowl since 1948, unranked, double-digit underdog UCLA defeated No. 4-ranked, Big Ten Champion Illinois 45-9 to win their second Rose Bowl in as many seasons.

"I couldn't really tell you what happened," said Illinois defensive tackle Mark Butkus—nephew of Illinois and Chicago Bears legend, Dick Butkus—but the score didn't begin to explain the football world's shock. In an ingenious bit of trickery, students from nearby engineering Xanadu, Cal Tech, had broken into the stadium and rewired the ancient scoreboard to switch from reading "Illinois" and "UCLA" to "MIT" and "Cal Tech" in the fourth quarter, prompting Illinois head coach Mike White, a California transplant, to declare, "The only highlight for me was when the scoreboard when out. It eased the pain a little."

Many of the 103,217 fans in attendance marveled at the amazing technical expertise of the pranksters, but even more were amazed that Don didn't capture his second MVP. He tied the Rose Bowl single-game record with two interceptions, both in the first quarter. Combined with his 1982 theft against Michigan, Don had set the career record for Rose Bowl game interceptions with three. He recorded 15 tackles, many of them punishing, and almost single-handedly shut down the California-grown, University of Illinois quarterback-receiver combo of Jack Trudeau and two-time All-America wide receiver David Williams, who, after a few early Don Rogers hits, proceeded to drop several passes inside "Mr. Rogers' neighborhood."

Though Don dominated from start to finish—more spectacularly, even, than the year before—UCLA quarterback Rick

THE ALL-AMERICA TRAGEDY OF DON ROGERS

Neuheisel won MVP. Neuheisel, who had the same bout of food poisoning that had kept two of his teammates from playing, was 22-for-31 for 288 yards and four touchdowns. As Don knew well from high school, quarterbacks usually have more impact on games than safeties. But as far as defense goes, it's a safety's impact on receivers that matters. And after the first quarter, sometime before the ingenious Cal Tech prank, Illinois star David Williams seemed terrified to catch the ball anywhere near Don Rogers.

The morning after the game, Tracy Dodds of *The Los Angeles Times*, a frequent Rogers interviewer, began her article with, "Don Rogers speaks softly. It's one of the scariest things about him."

The Illinois players would probably disagree.

Don became a consensus All-American, winning every award the Pac-10 offers. He was selected for the Hula Bowl and Japan Bowl All-Star games as well, and as the first player in UCLA to record three straight 100-tackle seasons, Don finished second on the school's all-time list with 409—behind Philadelphia Eagles All-Pro linebacker Jerry Robinson. He also finished third in career interceptions, and because Don spent his freshman year backing up iron-man Kenny Easley, he achieved most of his statistics in three seasons.

A partial list of first-team All-America team honors includes Football Coaches, Football Writers, Walter Camp, *Playboy*, *The Sporting News*, *Football News*, *College* and *Pro Football Weekly*, as well as notice from AP, UPI and NEA. He had been UCLA's MVP, team captain, MVP of the USC game, *Los Angeles Times* Player of the Year, and recipient of dozens of other awards and honors that were both obscure and famous, big and small.

After everything that had transpired in the past four years, including the birth of his son and his own rise to stardom, Don now had to prepare for the 1984 NFL draft. A few weeks after the Rose Bowl, Gayland Houston signed a Letter of Intent to play his college football at the University of California-Berkeley, a member of the Pac-10 Conference.

ONE MOMENT CHANGES EVERYTHING

❖ ❖ ❖

While Don steadily ascended to even bigger things, Reggie and Jackie were beginning to falter.

Up in Seattle, Reggie had gone from Pac-10 freshman of the year to splitting time his sophomore season with newly arrived 7-foot freshman center Christian Welp from Holland. Reggie may not have been happy with his "demotion," but Washington fans were ecstatic. Suddenly, the Huskies had become a player on the national college hoops scene. Reggie averaged 8.4 points and 5.3 rebounds a game as Washington won the Pac-10; but Detlef Shrempf, another European import, was the star of that team, which went 24-7, finished No. 15 in the nation, and defeated Mike Krzyzewski's first NCAA tournament team at Duke, a squad comprised of Jay Bilas, Mark Alarie, Johnny Dawkins, and Tommy Amaker. After the season, Huskies head coach Marv Harshman was named the NCAA Coach of the Year.

Reggie made no secret of his frustration over splitting playing time, and Coach Harshman, an old-school disciplinarian, made no secret of his contempt for anything that hindered his team's chemistry or winning. Still, Reggie seethed as Christian Welp got the minutes at center.

He now stood a shade under 6-foot-7 and weighed 235 pounds, and because his rim-rattling dunks and prowess for pulling down tough rebounds in traffic had made him one of the most intimidating players in the country, Reggie was now cast as the Huskies bruiser. Being an enforcer was not what Reggie had in mind when, just over a year earlier, he and Ernest Lee had ended every conversation with the phrase, "See you in the NBA!"

Although he was not the team's star, not yet, Reggie still had his moments of greatness on the court. He had a good game in the win over Duke, hitting four-of-five shots and pulling down half a dozen rebounds, all of which were integral in the two-point win that sent the Blue Devils back to Durham and put Washington in the Sweet 16. But with Welp only a freshman, Reggie's relationship with Harshman eroded, and he thought he saw the writing on the wall. He may have, on some level, blamed Harshman's favoritism for his demotion, but Reggie was growing up in other ways, and he was determined to be a star.

Two hundred miles south of Seattle, in Corvallis, Oregon, Jackie, a freshman who by now stood 6-foot-2 and was slated to start at forward for OSU, was finding life away from Del Paso Heights more difficult than she'd imagined. She didn't like the small town, and the lack of enthusiasm for basketball that had begun to arise during her last year of high school had followed her to college.

Cheryl Miller aside, women's college hoops of the early 1980s, even at the highest levels, was not an aesthetically pleasing game. Physically, women would make some of the biggest strides in sports history in the 1980s. Still, so little was thought of female athleticism that an archaic women's rule for basketball prohibited more than three players from either team from crossing half court at the same time. As of 1983, too few great female players existed to stimulate fan interest unless those fans had a strong connection to the college or university. Women's games, even the NCAA Championship, were seldom televised, and most universities had no following whatsoever. Under coach Aki Hill, Oregon State had been a women's NCAA championship contender for years; but away from Norte, her brothers, and her mother, Jackie didn't feel the connection or urgency necessary to excel.

Talent, however, was certainly not an issue.

A properly motivated Jackie Rogers could have played for any school in America. Incredibly, after just one season, and much to her family's dismay, Jackie, always the sole resident of her own ethereal world, without warning, resigned her scholarship, and quit the Oregon State basketball team.

Loretha was furious—and she was equally distressed that Reggie was in a funk over his diminishing role with the Huskies, which had caused him to neglect his studies and put him in danger of flunking out of school. With the three children dispersed across the West Coast, she was sensing, for the first time, the precarious state of their emotions. Luckily for everyone, they had Donald.

ONE MOMENT CHANGES EVERYTHING

Don would take care of Reggie, Jackie, and his son, Little D. Don would take care of everyone. If Jackie really wanted to drop out of Oregon State, then he would cover the cost of her classes at nearby Sacramento State. If losing his starting spot was the real reason that Reggie was depressed and failing, then Don had the idea that inexorably altered the direction of his brother's life, when he convinced Reggie to call the UW football coach, Don James, to see if he could try out for the team.

Right then and there, a light went off for Reggie: He'd show Harshman and anyone who had ever doubted him. He'd show everyone just what he could do.

Amidst the challenges and changes, the most glorious news to date came to the Rogers family. Don Rogers was selected by the Cleveland Browns with the 18th pick of the first round of the 1984 NFL draft.

Browns fans, who knew exactly what Don had done to the previous two seasons' Big Ten champions—Michigan and Illinois—rejoiced. Cleveland's head coach, Sam Rutigliano, a charismatic, old-school, working-class coach, instantly anointed Don the starting free safety for a team that already boasted a hard-hitting defense.

Suddenly, Don was rich, which meant the Rogers family was rich, too. He signed a three-year, $2.5 million contract and immediately bought his mother a house in a new development in South Natomas, which, although on the "safe" side of the tracks, was still a short, ominous walk away from Strawberry Manor.

8

Today, many Sacramento Kings players make their homes in the neighborhood of Los Lagos. Located in the Sierra Foothills near Folsom Lake and about 20 minutes from downtown Sacramento, the neighborhood is predominantly white, but black, Asian, and Arab millionaires live amongst the multitude of mansions as well. Los Lagos didn't exist when Don signed his first contract. Yet, in 1984 America, the actions of a 22-year-old African American seemed disparate compared to today's bonus babies, who call a realtor as soon as the ink on their contracts is dry and are met by limos waiting to show them their cavernous new homes with five-car garages.

Don now had the ability to purchase a house for his mother—which was a house for himself—anywhere in Sacramento. A grown man since youth, Don had been called upon to be a man for so many years; yet when the time came, he still felt compelled to live where he felt most comfortable. Or perhaps Loretha had insisted.

But why not move to the hills around town? Why not escape the urban life and set up house on the bluffs high above the Sacramento or American rivers?

While any number of reasons could explain why Don may have wanted to stick close to his roots, none involved posses or keeping it real. Don wouldn't have known a posse if he'd been a sheriff in a small western town. The reality is, he had known just two homes in his young life: the Rogers' Del Paso Heights shack and the UCLA campus.

ONE MOMENT CHANGES EVERYTHING

Though both offered insulation from the realities awaiting many young black men in the inner city, even if Don had been more comfortable, it's safe to say that Loretha would've wanted to stay close to where she called home. After all, this was a woman who had experienced real racial discrimination, who was always on the lookout for injustice—perceived or otherwise—and who lived in a city that had been included on a recent list of America's most segregated urban areas.

One of the new home's advantages was its proximity to Robertson Community Center, where Don and Reggie would lift weights and play ball with the kids. Also, the house was closer to Little D's mother. Simply, Del Paso Heights was Don's 'hood, and apparently he never gave moving away a second thought.

Characteristically, the next thing Don did with his money was organize and sponsor a children's flag-football league. He paid for all the equipment and hired the officials. For the older kids, Don, with Reggie's help, founded a new Pop Warner team. Their mascot? The Browns.

Grades and responsibility became mantric staples of the programs; and before they could join the Rogers' Browns, prospective players had to bring their report cards and notes from their teachers attesting to their good behavior. Though children may not always listen to their parents or teachers, professional football players tend to impose larger-than-life influence, so of course the kids wanted to improve their grades—even if only because Don Rogers told them to do so. Arguments arose over who would wear Don's No. 20 jersey. He was royalty to them, and finally a mandate had to be instituted so that a new player could wear his number each week. Soon, Browns jerseys were all over North Sacramento, and if you drove past a playground, you would see no less than half a dozen kids wearing Don's No. 20.

As could be expected, challenges arose along with the extreme changes in Don's life. A young man raised in poverty, he suddenly had money to spare—something that tests the natures of even the strongest individuals. Don bought his brother and sister a car each, then purchased stepfather Joe Henry a new Cadillac—which Joe still has.

"But then everyone came with their hands out," said longtime friend and coach, Dale Burney, the type of man that often worked three jobs to make ends meet and now lives in a beautiful home—albeit still in Del Paso Heights. Earlier that same year, 1984, Burney and his new wife had spent a portion of their honeymoon visiting Don at UCLA. "After he signed his contract, everyone wanted money."

Suddenly having a safety net where a bottomless pit had lurked previously encourages many to be reckless—but not Don, who still needed a few courses to graduate and arranged to attend summer school back in Los Angeles. Yet that statement was true for others, namely Joe Henry, who drove his new car straight to jail after being arrested twice for drunk driving in the 12 months that followed. A third such arrest two years later sent him to jail for 120 days.

The destroyed lives of lottery winners are well documented. Don would not end up owing more money than he made—and he was definitely not flashy—but he did have some friends who still struggled between sink and swim. It was, after all, The Heights, and Don was only four years out of high school; so friends soon came looking for money to pay the rent, or feed their addictions. Don said yes to as many as he could, but not because he wanted to be revered. He was already the most loved and worshiped man in town. And being that he was, as much as anyone truly is, self-made and had worked hard for his success, if he said "no" to any request, he did so with good reason.

Before Don's junior year at UCLA, he had fallen in love with a deacon's daughter named Leslie Nelson. Star running back Kevin Nelson—no relation to Leslie—had introduced the two. When Don had finished his senior season of football, Leslie had already become part of the Rogers family, and Don part of hers. She was close to Little D, and though they were only 22 years old, Don and Leslie became engaged. Their relationship was so strong that Leslie would often stay at the Rogers' new house, even when Don was away.

ONE MOMENT CHANGES EVERYTHING

With a brother preparing to embark on a pro football career, Reggie Rogers suddenly became serious about his own future. He too desired the wider benefits of being a star athlete. To anyone outside of fame, all fame seems grand, like its own reward. That reward is so in demand that late-night promises are made in soon-forgotten prayers, claiming that no further pleas will be made so long as the request for fame is granted. But college fame doesn't pay the rent or keep you warm at night. High school superstar? Check. College star? Check. While certain family members seemed more than willing to allow Don's wealth to support them—forever, if necessary—Reggie's suddenly realized that the only limitations on his talent were his own. Don had broken through, and momentum was still on the family's side. Now was Reggie's time to find his own way as well.

Their ticket, though, was athletics, and in that realm, Reggie always had coasted more than Don. In fact, his impressive size allowed Reggie to coast and still dominate. He had been bigger than other kids for his entire life; and, as his insistence to play JV basketball when he could've contributed alongside Don demonstrates, Reggie had the desire—if not a subconscious need—to dominate.

But how would Reggie respond when he could no longer dominate on size alone? Would he rise to the occasion, work hard? Or would he, as Jackie appeared to be doing, simply fade away into obscurity?

As a basketball player for Washington, Reggie was good—though he hadn't come close to reaching his immense potential. He was strong and fearsome and his rim-rattling dunks were favorites of Husky fans, but they also served to intimidate opponents.

But in its way, dunking is but a sideshow. And besides, Coach Harshman obviously favored the 7-foot freshman Christian Welp, in part, no doubt, because he was easier to coach, which, as his own long career wound down, mattered a great deal to Marv Harshman. Harshman had cut his teeth in a time when character, which meant that players listened to people in authority, mattered above all else.

THE ALL-AMERICA TRAGEDY OF DON ROGERS

Reggie wanted to play more at forward, which would seem natural for a player a shade under 6-foot-7; but he was a wide body in a skinny era who could take up space in the key. Harshman liked the idea of bringing Reggie off the bench to bang and wear down the opposition's 7-footers. And despite his breakout freshman season, Harshman's teams were stocked with enough talent and future pros that he didn't feel starting Reggie was necessary.

Reggie wasn't ready to give up basketball, which truly was his passion; and his place on the team was the beautiful bird in his giant hand. But he did want to sniff the football garden. What if he had sold himself short three years before? What if he truly was a natural? If Harshman wouldn't let him be a star, then maybe Don James would allow him to "break through." If history is any indicator, Reggie wouldn't have wanted to heap any further expectations or additional pressure upon himself. Outwardly, he simply wanted to see if he could hack college football.

But inwardly, it's more likely that Reggie was scared to death. He was used to stardom and was from a family of stars. People around Del Paso Heights expected a lot from Don's little brother. Dominance wasn't just easy for him—it was the norm that fed something inside Reggie's soul. Dominance satiated the hunger inside him that all young people share, but which some find harder to satisfy than others. Reggie just had more and more trouble feeling full.

Aside from an injury or foul trouble, Reggie had never sat on a bench, anywhere, anytime, or for any other reason. An All-Pac-10 freshman team member and serious candidate for the upcoming Olympic team, suddenly Reggie was no longer a starter on a good, but not yet great Huskies squad. This could not be happening.

This was severe stress for a 20-year-old icon—and it couldn't have been easy.

Issues of his brother's greatness would always surround Reggie. Don may or may not have felt a rivalrous friction between he and his brother, but that seems unlikely given Don's personality. Too few among mortals can compete with such a pristine presence living across the hall, though, and the affinity of complete strangers was a constant reminder of how Reggie didn't match up, no matter what he'd accomplished. He had branched off to play basketball in the Pacific Northwest, a thousand miles away from his brother. For whatever the reason—a bad coach, Ernest Lee's exodus, whatever—by his own lofty standards, Reggie was failing.

For all those who have faced adversity, the question is how they will respond.

People had begun to doubt Reggie, who was determined not to be ordinary, not to become just another face on the Washington campus. God forbid, he would be remembered in The Heights as nothing more than Don Rogers' little brother. He had to show those watching, including basketball coach Marv Harshman—whose patience with Reggie was paper thin—that they all needed him. As the cracks in his shaky foundation began to show, the football tryout was becoming the paramount crux of his young life, and success would be his spackle.

Yet, Washington didn't need gimmicks or outsiders to save the day. Year in and year out, Washington was one of the top producers of NFL talent, and a record 11 players had been chosen in the 1983 draft alone. They had gone to the 1981 and 1982 Rose Bowls and five straight bowl games overall. The Huskies were known for tough scheduling and even tougher wins. On any given day, they could beat any school in the nation. The 1982 Huskies finished 10-2, handing Don and Rose Bowl champion UCLA their only loss of the year. Washington was a deep, fast, tradition-rich team that for years had its pick of the Northwest's best recruits, including California.

Success notwithstanding, serious athletes just don't appreciate outsiders treating their passion as a hobby. A hark back to Michael Jordan's foray into baseball proves that. Many pitchers were dying to bean him, and ample animosity arose from players whose spots were threatened by his presence. Baseball didn't need Jordan, and the Huskies football team didn't need Reggie Rogers, either. He may have been big and bad and strong, but pushing around 180-pound "twigs" on the hardwood was hardly the same as taking on 300-pound behemoths from Ohio State and Michigan.

THE ALL-AMERICA TRAGEDY OF DON ROGERS

However, Reggie was no ordinary physical specimen. So when he showed up for his first practice, curious coaches who had wanted him for football three years earlier were still looking for the next great thing. Some full-time football players, though—themselves proud athletes—definitely wanted to see Reggie Rogers get knocked on his ass.

To make matters more compelling, Don Rogers' second choice for college was to play for Don James at Washington. The family ties, the name recognition, Reggie's status on campus—this wasn't just any big body coming to screw around with a football, this guy's brother had been the best of them all.

Still, when Reggie showed up for the first day of practice, Huskies players viewed his supposed talent and the difficult transition with cynicism. Reggie hadn't worn pads for almost three years, and the last time he'd played a game—the riot at Winters High School—had ended in defeat and injury.

The Huskies coaches, who weren't looking for a sideshow, didn't mince words or waste time, throwing Reggie headfirst into the ring. He was grouped with the outside linebackers, and instead of agility or passing drills to let him get his feet wet, they set up a *mano-a-mano* tackling drill where the ball carrier had to run full throttle right at the defender.

As Reggie approached his turn in line, he faced a daunting reality: He hadn't tackled anyone in years. Worse yet, he had *never* tackled anyone with the size and speed of a Washington tailback. Besides, tackling in practice is, in many ways, more difficult than tackling in actual games. Game tackling is instinctual and takes place within a vacuum of desperation and opportunity. Jerseys, ankles, necks, and legs—anything and everything—are fair game so long as the defender stops the ball carrier in games. Tackling someone in practice is another matter. In practice, a player is expected to use perfect form, overcoming head-on angles in an unnatural scenario that rarely presents itself in actual games. To make matters more difficult, all running backs become power backs in drills—there's no touchdown to score, and reputations for toughness are at stake. The tackler is required to stay up high to avoid injury. Moreover, the tailback isn't allowed to stop, make moves, or juke. It's a tackling drill. It's about proving one's mettle. And it's as staged and as unnatural as Sumo wrestlers colliding with a 20-yard sprint to muster a head of steam.

Everyone on campus knew Reggie, who was more visible on the basketball court than any football player at Husky Stadium. He had played great in the previous season's watershed NCAA Tournament victory over Duke, and certainly everyone on that field knew who Don Rogers was—his Rose Bowl resume had made him an icon on the West Coast. But if Reggie failed, or got run over, no doubt 100 players would immediately think, "Stick to basketball—you ain't your brother." Or perhaps everyone realized that Reggie had donned a helmet because his career in high tops was abating.

In any event, the entire Washington team knew why the tackling drill came before anything else for Reggie. So when Reggie took position for his turn, the usual practice-field activity stopped, just like an E.F. Hutton commercial. Everyone leaned closer to watch and listen. Even head coach Don James—with his CEO aura and a face that finished runner-up for Mt. Rushmore—joined the dozen assistant coaches and the 100-odd players studying the drill.

Reggie might have had a lump in his throat, but the throng of interested spectators probably made him feel right at home as the center of attention. Whatever Reggie did had always interested people. That part had to feel good, even though, simultaneously, it probably scared the hell out of him.

Ball in hand, the tailback ran parallel to the line of orange cones, looking for his opportunity to burst through as Reggie shuffled his feet awkwardly, trying to mirror the runner. For whatever reason, for no reason, the tailback picked his spot and suddenly wheeled upfield, dirt flying up behind his cleats. Gathering speed, he ran directly at the towering Reggie, making no effort to go wide or take a sweep angle. Seeing the runner barreling toward him, Reggie squatted down awkwardly like a quarterback taking a snap from his center, trying to get as low as possible. As the two met in a jolting helmet-to-helmet collision, in a blur of instincts and strength, Reggie somehow wrestled the ball carrier to the ground. His adrenaline pumping, infused with confidence, Reggie jumped to his feet, only to hear several Washington players laughing at him.

Reggie had tackled the back the only way he knew how. He had squatted in the "hole" between the cones, and waited for the runner to reach him. When they met, despite the running back's momentum and forward lean, Reggie gave up no ground—not even an inch. In fact, he stopped the runner cold, stood him up, corralled his legs, picked him up, and drove him into the ground, just as he was taught to do back in high school.

The players may have been laughing at Reggie's unnatural form, but the coaches weren't laughing at all. They'd seen all they needed. Reggie was tough. To stand his ground while a 220-pound fullback tried to flatten him required incredible natural strength. Instantly, half a dozen grown men in purple polo shirts muttered amongst themselves excitedly. At that moment, Reggie convinced them that he was talented and strong, and that he could make up for his three years away from the game. Unable to hide their excitement, the coaches descended on him with a million instructions and 76-rpm advice.

Reggie absorbed everything, listening intently, but he knew that he needed an expert to help him. Though he would have no trouble covering the field or making desperation tackles, he needed someone to coach him on the finer points of gridiron obliteration—on the geometry and physiology of impact, on the mental components of a game that he barely understood. In short, he needed a master, a professional hitter.

He needed Don.

The moment that the Huskies reached the locker room, Reggie was on the phone to his brother. ("I had to wait over an hour to use the pay phone," remembered star quarterback, Chris Chandler.) That evening, Don and Reggie spoke again. Don kept repeating to Reggie the most important aspect of tackling his way: hit through the ball carrier.

ONE MOMENT CHANGES EVERYTHING

"Hit through him. Hit him like he's standing 20 yards away."

Don's mantra worked for Reggie the same way it made sense to him that you dunk a basketball as hard as you possibly can. Reggie didn't just dunk the ball until his wrists touched the rim—he dunked through it, he tried to pull it down. The result pleased crowds and probably helped Reggie channel anger that otherwise would've swallowed him whole. But for now, there was football to be played. And Don James, who ranked nationally in the top ten for coaches' winning percentage, didn't win nearly 70 percent of his games by being an average judge of talent. Bloodlines, size, strength, and quickness made Reggie Rogers a marvel, and everyone could see it.

So as Don was beginning his rookie year in the NFL, Reggie was starting his rookie year of college football as well.

The results for both were outstanding.

9

Though the 1984 season had been tough, Cleveland fans still had reason to be optimistic, as their franchise seemed to be compiling all the pieces of a winner. After a 1-7 start featuring several close losses, ownership replaced the popular, but ineffective head coach, Sam Rutigliano, with Pennsylvania native Marty Schottenheimer—a man who seemed born to lead a NFL franchise. The Browns went just 4-4 in the second half, but with Chip Banks, Clay Matthews, Handford Dixon, and Don Rogers, the team finished No. 1 in the league in total defense, thrilling the Cleveland Dawg Pound—who may be the best dressed and most loyal fans in the game. While the Browns had holdover stalwarts, such as future Hall of Fame tight end Ozzie Newsome, the premier tight end in football, the team's pulse was young and aggressive.

The difference between Division I football and the NFL is exponential, far greater than the leap from high school to college ball and perhaps the greatest jump in any sport. But that didn't faze Don, whose hard-hitting play immediately made him a Cleveland fan favorite. Despite a mid-season shoulder separation that forced him to miss a game, Don scintillated throughout his rookie season. He was the kind of safety who caused more fumbles and dropped passes than one who accumulates high interception numbers. Possessing impeccable timing, he would routinely arrive at the same instant as the pass; and even if the receiver managed to hang on to the ball, he paid a terrible price—often resulting in a drop on the next one, or the one after that.

ONE MOMENT CHANGES EVERYTHING

When his rookie season had ended, Don had finished fourth on the Browns in tackles behind the three starting linebackers, two of which, USC graduates Chip Banks and Clay Matthews, were coming off Pro Bowl seasons. For his performance over the course of the 1984 season the NFL Players Association elected Don as the AFC Defensive Rookie of the Year—meaning that the veteran players around the league chose Don from a pool of over 200 drafted players and several hundred more who signed as free agents as the top rookie defender in the AFC. He was also voted to the UPI, *Pro Football Weekly*, *Football Digest*, and *Professional Football Writers Association* all-rookie teams. With Lott, Easley, Dennis Smith, and others, this was the golden age for safeties in the NFL—and journalists, coaches, and players alike saw Don as the NFL's next great defensive back.

One of Don's rookie-year highlights came in the very first game of the regular season. The Browns had traveled to Seattle to face the Seahawks, where he would get to play against his close friend Kenny Easley, as well as see his brother, Reggie, who had gone from preseason curiosity to starting outside linebacker for the Huskies. (The Seahawks dominated the season-opening game with Cleveland, winning 33-0. A day earlier, the Huskies destroyed Northwestern 26-0, giving Seattle a sweep of the visiting Midwestern teams.)

Despite his time away from the game and the steep learning curve of a new position, Reggie embarked upon his new challenge and would also enjoy a huge season. Perhaps second only to the 1990 national championship team, the 1984 Washington Huskies may have been the best team in school history. While Reggie was often required to drop into pass coverage from his linebacker position, the coaches loved his potential as a pure pass rusher. He recorded 74 tackles, five sacks, forced three fumbles, and knocked down three passes in his first football season in three years, earning the team's Most Improved Player award.

Reggie's phenomenal athletic abilities, superior to most of his peers, allowed him to shake off three years of rust and start for one of college football's top programs. He used his size and agility to wreak havoc from sideline to sideline. Just like Hall of Fame defensive end Hugh Green, Reggie's speed helped him track down unsuspecting ball carriers on opposite-end sweeps and lock them up with his 7-foot wingspan. He was never so much a great football or basketball player as he was a dominant athlete who could meld his talents to any physical endeavor. But could Reggie improve? Would he improve?

The Huskies finished the 1984 regular season 10-1. As UCLA prepared for the Fiesta Bowl and USC for the Rose Bowl, Washington was scheduled to meet heavily favored Oklahoma—and its new-age media creation, linebacker Brian Bosworth—in the Orange Bowl. Yet, in what would become a troubling pattern, something happened off the field that overshadowed preparation for the game. A dust up between Reggie and Bosworth at a pre-Orange Bowl party may have been the most telling example of Reggie's hair-trigger state of mind.

Or perhaps Brian Bosworth deserved it. ...

At a cruise ship media event to honor both teams, some Washington players were in a club area listening to music, when in walked The Boz and some Oklahoma teammates, intent on making their presence felt. Either Bosworth truly hated the music or he simply wanted to make a scene, but he marched directly to the DJ and demanded that he play country music. When the DJ refused, Bosworth made the change himself.

With country music warbling throughout the club, the Huskies' festive mood was quelled. Stunned, they watched as Boz strutted to their table and stood in front of Reggie, who was talking with a few teammates. A forerunner to Dennis Rodman and Terrell Owens on the "me-first" carousel ride—a never-ending, thrill-a-minute experience that gives and takes in equal measure—Bosworth had found his target.

To his credit, at least this time, Bosworth was picking on someone his own size. After a stare off that would have made Apollo Creed blanch, Boz suddenly leapt upon the small cocktail table, and standing above Reggie and looking down, he started performing an exaggerated, mocking "ho-down" dance, complete with boot heel-clicking and thumbs hooked into his imaginary suspenders.

Now, Reggie was from The Heights, where indecision could get a person killed just as fast as rising to take the bait. No matter, Reggie liked to get active. He cleanly kicked the table from beneath Bosworth, whose cowboy boots landed with a smack on the dance floor. Surrounded by their respective teams, the two players faced off in a scene that threatened to become riotous.

Though a few half-hearted punches were thrown on the periphery, order was quickly restored when Don James and the Washington coaches arrived unexpectedly. In a scene straight of Doc's candy store in *West Side Story*, just as the rival gangs Jets and Sharks had, the adversaries pretended to be best friends so that no one in authority would realize what had happened. Had he known, no doubt Don James immediately would have suspended everyone involved. Whether a rumble beneath the freeway—or in this case under the docks—was planned to follow is unclear, but no further extracurricular flare-ups were reported.

Washington went on to win the Orange Bowl 28-17, and finish the year ranked No. 1 in the country by *Football News* and the *Chicago Tribune*, and No. 2 in virtually every other poll. For the fourth year in a row, Washington had spent at least some stretch of time as the No. 1-ranked team in the country. Along with UCLA's 39-37 Fiesta Bowl win over Miami and USC's 20-17 victory over Ohio State in the Rose Bowl, the Pac-10 Conference earned national bragging rights with wins in three of the four (the Sugar Bowl being the other) major New Year's Day bowl games.

In less than a year, Reggie had led Washington to a win over Duke in the NCAA basketball tournament and had established himself as a rising star in an Orange Bowl victory over Oklahoma—heady stuff for a 20-year-old. After only a single season, scouts already had their sights on him as a potential future NFL star, which was no doubt exciting for everyone in the Rogers family; but Reggie had a surprise for all of them.

He wasn't finished with basketball just yet.

THE ALL-AMERICA TRAGEDY OF DON ROGERS

Only hours after the Orange Bowl, Reggie was back at basketball practice and primed, not only to partake in what promised to be a great season, but determined to regain his starting position in the sport he loved best of all.

Whether Marv Harshman actually liked coaching Reggie is unknown. With the exception of Detlef Shrempf, Reggie admittedly didn't mix well with the other Huskies players. The old-school Harshman usually recruited a particular type of player, though—and character was foremost in his mind. His reports on the young Rogers were certainly positive, and since Don was Reggie's brother, some of his qualities were automatically assumed to be inherent in Reggie as well. Don was known in Pac-10 circles as a gentleman and a team player, someone who insisted that he was from a good family, and someone who always put his team first.

Perhaps Reggie's talent had blinded Harshman, but the coach still ran a clean program. Allegations had been thrown his way by Jerry Tarkanian, though, who accused him of "stashing" Ernest Lee—Reggie's running mate whose life ended in a tragic turn of events.

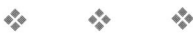

If the Rogers family had a Sacramento-area rival for basketball honors and media attention, Ernest Lee, who brought Pearl Washington's flair to the Capitol City game, was that player. Lee had dropped off the face of the earth after leaving Washington, though, and many expected the worst for the young man who seemed to have little else on his mind but basketball.

Ernest, however, surprised everyone. He reappeared on the college scene with a flashy vengeance. After leaving Seattle, Ernest traveled east to Atlanta to live with his mother. A chance encounter with Robert Pritchett, the highly regarded head coach at Atlanta's African-American Division II power, Clark College (now called Clark Atlanta College), earned Ernest a tryout. He started from that moment forward, and averaging over 30 points per game, he led the entire nation in scoring for three straight years—a remarkable achievement at any level.

In 1987, at the end of his senior season, Clark College retired Ernest Lee's No. 23 jersey. NBA scouts had attended many of his games, interviewed Ernest, and there was speculation that he would be a late-round draft pick. That was all Ernest needed—he knew that once he got the chance, he would make good in the NBA.

But NBA super scout Marty Blake didn't think the league had room for Lee, and he said so. Lee had spent much of his collegiate career playing forward for an undersized Division II team, sometimes against less-than-stellar competition. At 6-foot-3, Lee had been a spectacular high school point guard, but had he lost some of his handle playing forward in Atlanta?

Kevin Johnson thought so. "I really think he was a better player coming out of high school than he was coming out of Clark," said Johnson. "He was certainly better than me at the time. He was a trendsetter when Sacramento didn't set trends."

When "KJ," as Johnson is known, was selected with the No. 7 pick in the 1987 NBA draft, Lee's fate, if not his career, may have inadvertently been sealed. No one would wish the experience upon his worst enemy: Ernest Lee sitting in the Omni in Atlanta, watching the seven-round draft unfold, his fierce Sacramento Metro League rival selected with the seventh pick. Then Lee, intently focusing on the first syllable of each name of every pick, sat hoping to hear "Ernest" somewhere along the way.

Undrafted, Lee later walked the streets of the city, then went home and told his mother, "All I wanted to do was play ball, and they wouldn't let me. What am I going to do with the rest of my life?"

"It was devastating to me, too," said Pritchett, regarding his star player going undrafted.

Lee briefly played professionally in Europe, but came home to Sacramento, where he was an early cut by head coach Bill Russell and the now hometown Sacramento Kings, who had moved to the city in 1985.

THE ALL-AMERICA TRAGEDY OF DON ROGERS

The future would not be kind to Ernest Lee. He did construction work for a high school teammate's father and volunteered at a local youth ministry in South Sacramento, where everyone agreed that the children loved him, and he made life a little lighter with his—outwardly, at least—upbeat attitude and easy smile.

Seven years later, on January 10, 1994, Ernest Lee, in a pattern common to depressed people, went through the ritual of saying goodbye to his friends and family. He called his father in Mississippi, a man he hadn't spoken to in years. He phoned his mother in Atlanta, and then sent a favorite shirt to a niece who had always coveted the garment. Ernest then borrowed his grandmother's car and drove to the orange Capitol Bridge that spans the river in downtown Sacramento. Leaving no note, he scaled that clunky bridge. The city that once anointed him player of the year glowed brightly to his right, and the murky brown water rushed merlessly 100 feet below. Revered in both Sacramento and Atlanta, but not inside his own mind, for whatever reasons, Ernest Lee jumped to his death on a cold January night—the victim of everything and everyone, of nothing and no one, all at the same time.

It took a month to find Lee's body. Longtime rival Kevin Johnson, now an NBA All-Star averaging 20 points and 9.5 assists per game for Phoenix, helped organize and finance the funeral. A thousand people showed up to pay their last respects.

In 2006, the prestigious Sacramento Versus the Bay Area All-Star Basketball Tournament was dedicated to the memory of Ernest Lee. Kevin Johnson had been first choice among the organizers as honoree, but the administrators quickly decided that recognizing Johnson was too easy. Recognizing Ernest Lee, they decided, was the right thing to do, as Ernest had done his part to put Sacramento basketball on the map and had been the better high school player. Kevin Johnson, who during his 11-year NBA career averaged 20.0 points and 10.0 assists three different times (making him one of only four players in NBA history to do so), has enough money to live anywhere he chooses, but instead runs charter schools and

ONE MOMENT CHANGES EVERYTHING

ministries in Sacramento's notorious Oak Park neighborhood through the Kevin Johnson Foundation. When told of the committee's intention to honor Lee, Johnson insisted the administrators had made the correct choice. At this high school All-Star event in 2006, the circumstances surrounding Ernest Lee's life and death were employed to educate high school stars about the statistical realities of their some day playing in the NBA.

To this day, much bitterness unfortunately remains over Lee's broken dreams and ultimate demise. In the inner city, broken dreams of stardom are not uncommon; and as is sometimes the case, those closest to tragedy have the most difficulty making sense of the loss.

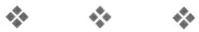

Some people assigned blame for Ernest Lee's demise to the man he went to Washington to learn from and never got the chance to play for—Marv Harshman. Due to Ernest's inability to handle the academics at UW, his academic probation prohibited his access to the basketball team's support system of trainers and tutors. Some people wonder if Marv Harshman should have ever recruited Ernest Lee in the first place.

Harshman, the last coach in NCAA history to defeat the great John Wooden in a game, retired after more than 40 years as a college coach at the end of the 1985 season—coincidentally, Reggie's last in a basketball uniform. Already in the NAIA Hall of Fame, Harshman was inducted into the NCAA Hall of Fame in April of that same year. But Harshman, whose career was interrupted so he could serve his country in World War II, would be the first to admit that he had trouble understanding the new generation of players. He was not adept at the "hand holding" that was required to ensure that adult men who were enrolled in college needed to be prodded to do what was in their own best interests for their futures: minor responsibilities such as going to class and studying hard.

THE ALL-AMERICA TRAGEDY OF DON ROGERS

A standout college player in the 1930s, Harshman began coaching in a time when the point of playing basketball wasn't to earn a shot at the NBA. Basketball was simply something a young man could utilize to help him get into college, which was considered the golden ticket to the good life in America. For Harshman, allowing a marginally qualified student such as Lee the opportunity to attend a university as prestigious as Washington should have been its own reward.

That wasn't enough for Ernest Lee; and it wasn't enough for Reggie, whose Washington basketball career had begun with the loftiest of expectations, but faced the danger of ending due to frustrating brawls and academic purgatory. As the 1985 basketball season wore down, Reggie, in his third year as a Huskies basketball player, had joined the team halfway through the season—and was now on the floor less than any time during the previous two years. Unhappy with the demotion, Reggie was in danger of becoming a disruption to the Washington basketball team.

Having ended only weeks before, Reggie's first season of playing Washington football had not been without controversy. Fans throughout the Pac-10 Conference were amazed by his fleet-footed athleticism, but they were equally startled by his vicious hits. Some of those hits came after the whistle—including one blindside shot that nearly snapped the head off Oregon quarterback Chris Miller, eliciting stunned gasps from fans genuinely surprised that Miller had been able to get up off the turf and walk away. Later in that same game, Reggie was assessed a penalty for a late hit on an Oregon running back.

Border supremacy, recruiting competition, and shared history combine to make the Universities of Oregon and Washington bitter rivals. In a scene reminiscent of Norte Del Rio's basketball games with Jesuit High—only now in front of 10,000 additional fans—Washington and Reggie traveled to Eugene for a Pac-10 basketball game against the Ducks that would determine first place in the conference.

Attending that evening were several Duck football players intent on exacting some verbal revenge on Reggie for his late hits;

but beyond that, how they expected to reach him was unclear. Reggie was now firmly entrenched on the Huskies bench, and only got to play in blowouts, or when center Christian Welp was in foul trouble.

For generations, Oregon's MacArthur Court has been voted as the Pac-10 conference's most difficult place to play. The 80-year-old bleachers crowd the court, making exchanges between fans and players inevitable. It gets loud, and Eugene, Oregon, is the spirited embodiment of a true "college town," where sellouts in football and basketball are common, and the fans live for the local team.

Oregon desperately needed the win to keep pace with the Huskies, who were far more talented. Behind Welp, silky forward Paul Fortier, and Detlef Shrempf, who played 16 NBA seasons, Washington had pulled away from the Ducks and were running their time-kill offense to preserve the important conference victory.

Late in the contest, Harshman inserted Reggie into the game for mop-up duty. Though Reggie seemed to be resigned to the end of his basketball career, his entrance into any game—in any town—magically incited crowds, who knew that a powerful dunk was on its way. At 250-plus pounds, with his knee braces and huge shoulders, Reggie didn't look like a college basketball player, either. Upon entering the game in Eugene, Reggie was taunted mercilessly by fans and Oregon football players, who had not forgiven his hit on Miller—nor where they thrilled about losing to conference rival Washington for the sixth straight time.

In an attempt to close the gap, Oregon applied a desperation full-court press. Reggie had caught the inbounds pass and was being bumped as much as guarded by an aggressive Oregon defender. A foul should have been called. Past injustices, the taunts of fans, the aggressive defender, the lack of playing time in his favored sport, and the end of his own personal hoop dreams all combined to ignite Reggie, who either used the ball or his forearm to shove the face of the defender, who slid several feet backwards across the MacArthur Court floor.

THE ALL-AMERICA TRAGEDY OF DON ROGERS

The fans went nuts. Debris rained down on the court, and while most of Oregon's basketball players may have been hesitant to challenge Reggie, football star Doug Judge was not.

In 1984-1985, Doug Judge was the captain of the Oregon football team and a respected figure around Eugene. He'd somehow managed to combine a rugged 6-foot-3 inch, 225-pound frame with a sprinter's speed to lead the entire nation in kickoff-return yardage. As Oregon's starting free safety, Judge was a big admirer of Don Rogers, and he knew a thing or two about hitting. He could not abide another Reggie cheap shot on an unprepared Oregon Ducks athlete.

When Judge leapt to his feet and began yelling at Reggie from his seat just a few rows off the court, Reggie may have motioned for the safety to come down and fight him. Judge hurdled the seats, and the two athletes—between them measuring nearly 13 feet in length and weighing almost 500 pounds—clashed before a partisan Oregon crowd.

Fortunately, a throng of players and security got between the two. Reggie was tossed from the game, and Judge reportedly was escorted from the building. However, Reggie now had cemented his reputation as intimidating and ill tempered: one that he would struggle to live down for many years to come. The question was: Would fans ever get to appreciate Reggie's remarkable athletic prowess, or would his future be defined by his lack of impulse control and anger?

After the game, Harshman, weary and just weeks away from the end of a highly decorated 40-year career spent coaching college basketball, evidently had had enough. Sometime later, when asked about Reggie's place as a basketball player at Washington, Harshman said only, "His future's in football."

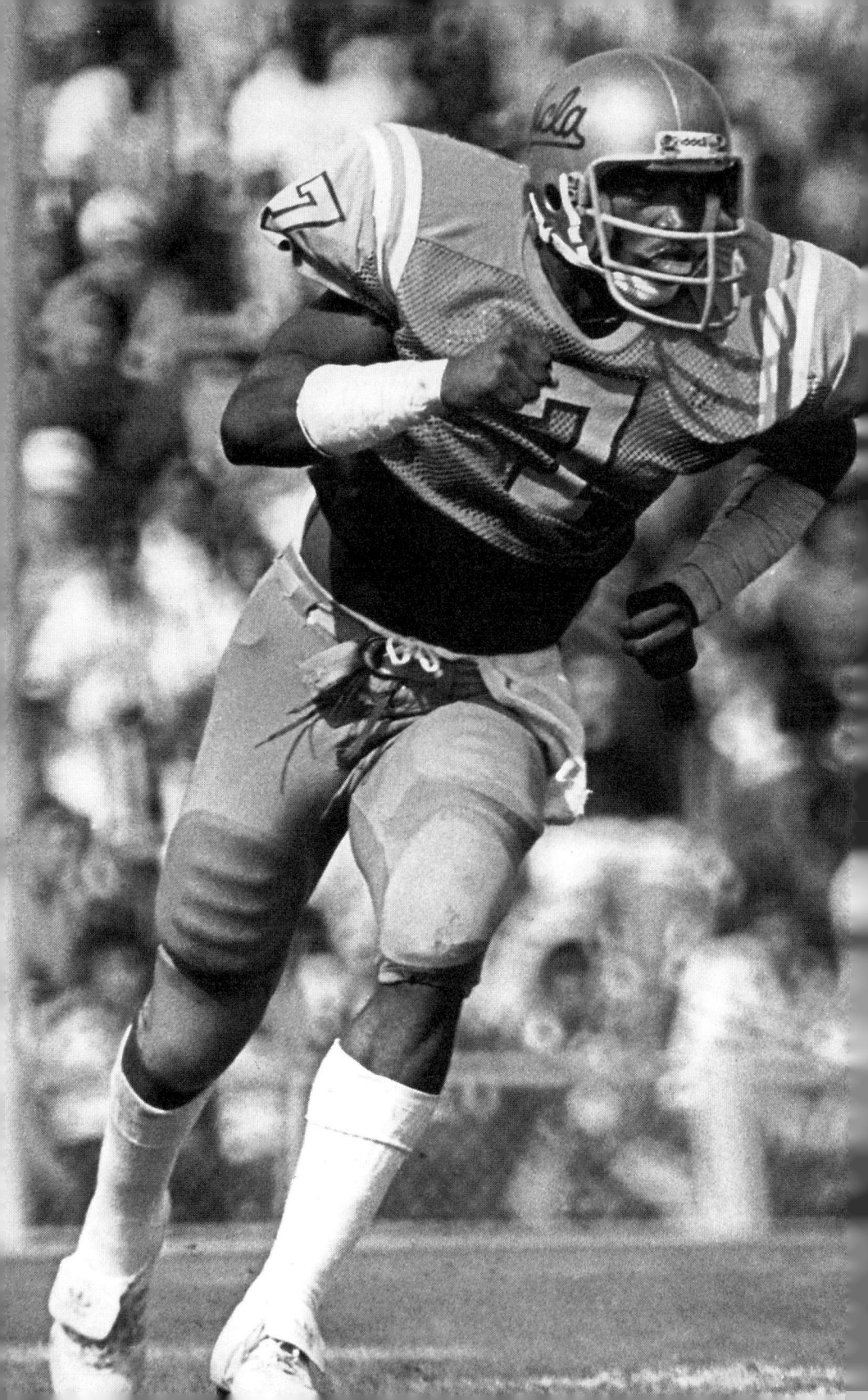

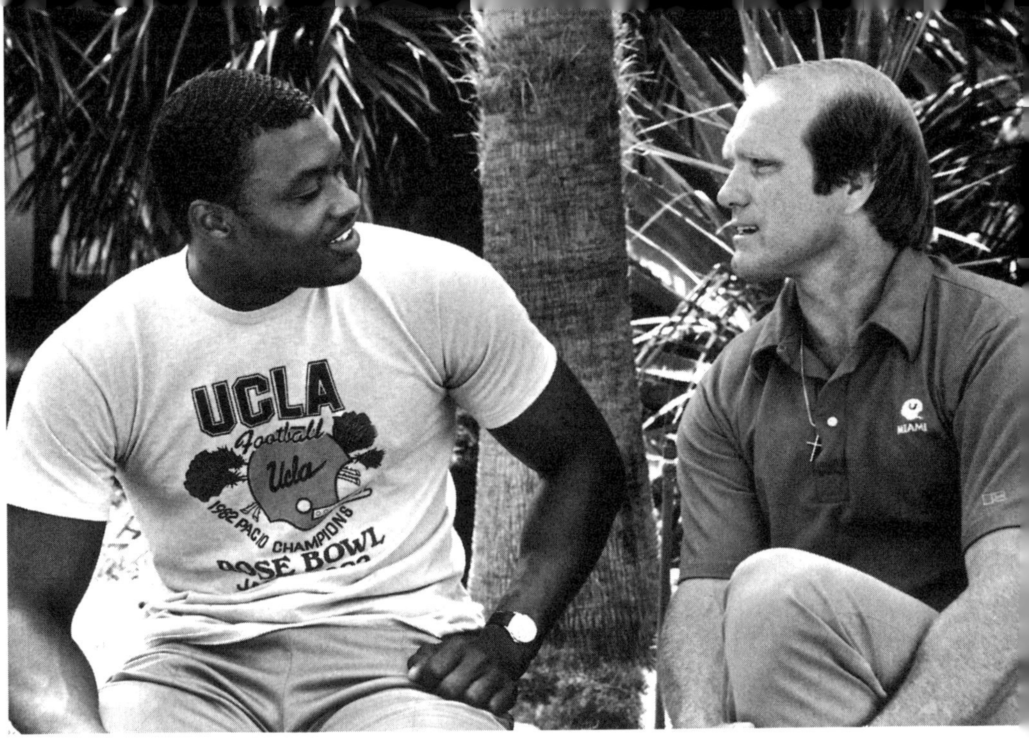

Left: Don Rogers (7) in action as a UCLA Bruin.
Above: Legendendary NFL quarterback Terry Bradshaw talks football with Don.
Below: A family friend weeps over Don Rogers' casket during his funeral service.
Photos courtesy of The Sacramento Bee
Following page: Don Rogers on the Cleveland Browns sideline in 1984.
Photo by George Gojkovich/Getty Images

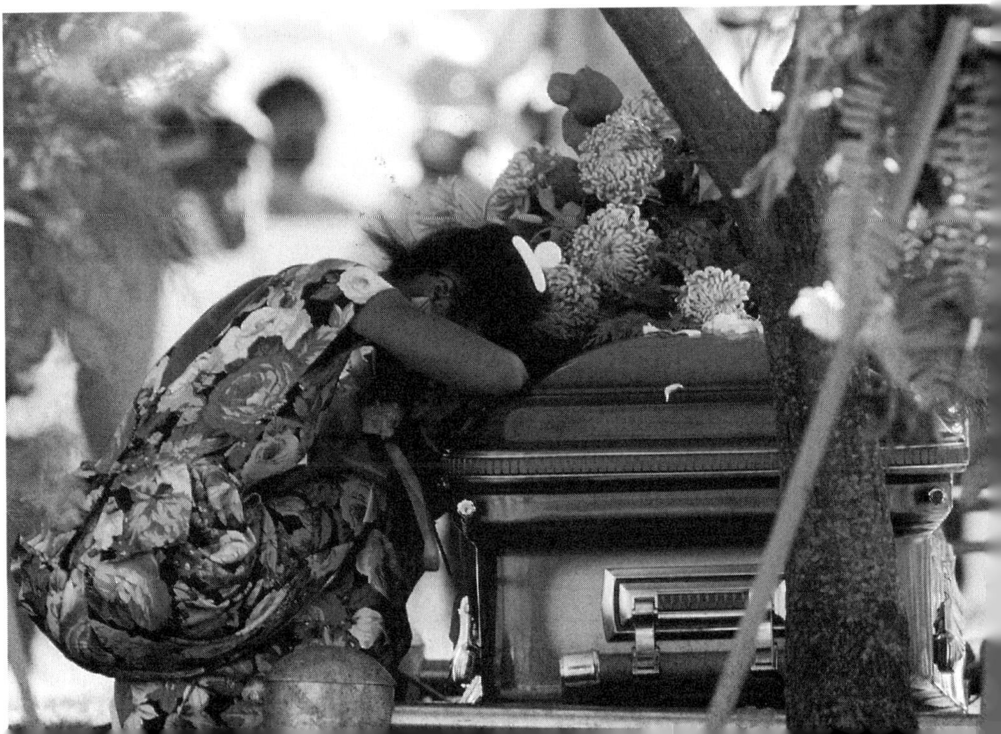

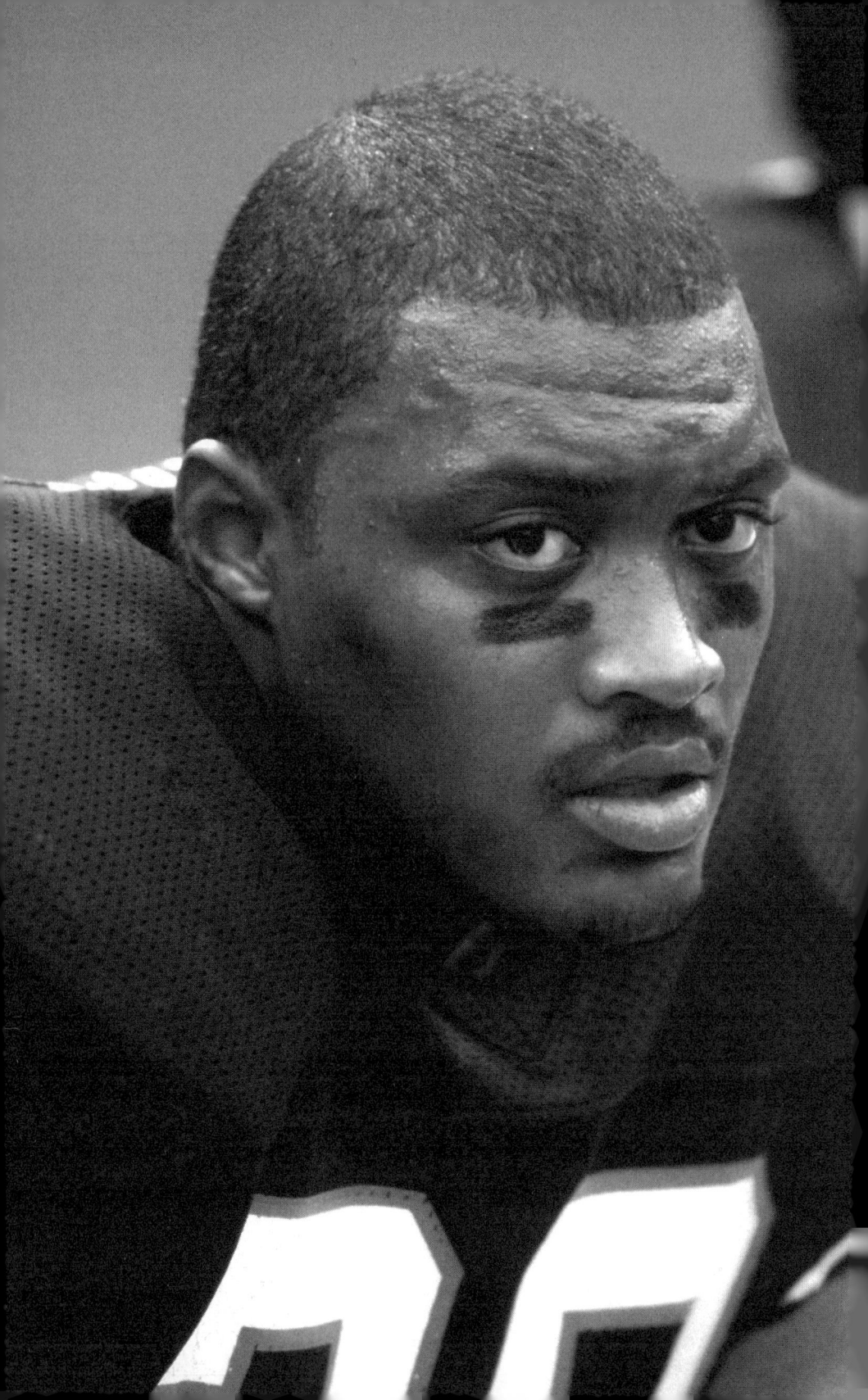

10

A pro football team's media guide is the best resource when searching for how a team truly feels about its players. Between "was everything the franchise had hoped for" and the dreaded "will have to improve," fans know where that player stands.

Heading into the 1985 season, the Cleveland Browns were more than pleased with the franchise's investments—especially its first-round draft pick from the previous year, Don Rogers. While football coaches strategically place quotes into their team's media guide to light a fire under certain players, that wasn't necessary with Don. The '85 Browns media guide contains a two-page homage to Don that reads like a fan website, proudly implying that the club made the perfect choice when they selected the former UCLA All-America safety.

Plucking quarterback Bernie Kosar from the University of Miami in the supplemental draft, then immediately implanting him as a starter suddenly thrust Cleveland into the NFL's elite. But the Browns were no offensive juggernaut. Built around their defense, on which Don Rogers was just one of five defensive starters chosen with first-round picks, the Browns punished offenses league-wide with tough guys and hard hitters at every position.

Playing in the rugged AFC Central division, Cleveland still managed to improve their record to 8-8, up from 5-11 the previous season. Four losses came by less than a touchdown. Yet, the team reaching the playoffs for just the second time in 14 years had fans excited.

ONE MOMENT CHANGES EVERYTHING

In their 24-21 playoff loss to the Miami Dolphins—a game in which the Browns took a 21-3 lead into the second half—Don intercepted a Dan Marino pass and returned it 45 yards to set up a 21-yard Earnest Byner touchdown dash that gave the Browns a 14-3 second-quarter lead.

In just his second professional season, Don had made the kind of leaps that characterized his UCLA career, where he'd gone from backup as a freshman to team leader in tackles as a sophomore, earning the Most Improved Player award. Don's sophomore year in the NFL was identical in that, after finishing fourth the year before, he led Cleveland in tackles with 154 (108 of which were solo stops), placing him almost 20 takedowns ahead of any teammate. With the exception of Seattle's Kenny Easley—and now Cleveland's Don Rogers—rarely did safeties lead the team in tackles. With only two years of experience, Don had gained a reputation among his peers as a fearless hitter and selfless team player; and everyone liked and respected him.

Having just completed the second year of his initial three-year contract, Don was in line for a big raise and long-term deal that would secure him and his family financially for years to come. He and Leslie, his college sweetheart, finalized their wedding plans as well: The date was set for June 28, 1986. Leslie's father would preside at his church in downtown Oakland.

With a potential guest list numbering over 500, the wedding sported Reggie as the best man, Kenny Easley and Don's teammate Hanford Dixon as ushers, and a roll call of future Hall of Fame inductees, former college standouts and coaches, and a long list of NFL stars. Of course, Little D would be the ring bearer in what was to be not only the "Wedding of the Year," but a golden opportunity to celebrate all Don had accomplished while preparing him for a future set in the brightness of the sun.

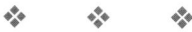

Reggie's junior year at Washington in 1985 revealed the new, more mature player and individual that everyone around him hoped he'd become. Whether his path to stardom was on track or he finally felt at peace with his place in the world is unclear, but coaches and teammates alike noticed a profound development, which translated into staggering on-field performances.

After the 1984 11-1 season, Reggie's first in football, the Huskies lost seven players to the NFL draft, including Ron Holmes, a defensive tackle taken in the first round by the Tampa Bay Buccaneers. Reggie was moved to defensive tackle, and while his height remained unchanged at just shy of 6-foot-7, he now weighed an imposing 260 solid and lightning-quick pounds—courtesy of those off-season workouts at Robertson with Don. The personnel losses forced Washington into a rebuilding year in which the Huskies finished 7-5—respectable, yet their worst season in nine years. Still, U-Dub did manage a 20-17 Freedom Bowl victory over Colorado that, though below program standards, allowed the bevy of underclassmen to gain valuable game experience, setting the stage for the following season.

Even though Jackie had inexplicably given up sports, the sun shone brightest on the Rogers family during this time. Somehow, after all the glory, their ascent to greatness surged even higher. What probably seemed unlikely to outsiders had happened: Reggie Rogers had become a bona fide college football superstar. Best of all, he had emerged as a hard-working and respected team leader. College sports offer a brief opportunity for success that an injury, bad attitude, or a coaching change can snuff out in a blink. Though a sense of urgency had found its way into Reggie, he also carried an obligation to his immense talent, something that he had previously taken for granted.

Reggie led the 1985 Huskies. Statistically, he led them in sacks with eight, in tackles along the defensive front with 112 (almost ten a game); and he recorded 15 stops of running backs for loss (second best in the Pac-10).

As the year progressed, Reggie improved; and by season's end, opponents could not block him one on one. An article ran in *The Los Angeles Times* that became part of the Reggie Rogers (and family) lore. UCLA coach Terry Donahue was watching film of the

ONE MOMENT CHANGES EVERYTHING

Bruins' upcoming opponent and couldn't take his eyes off a dominating defensive tackle. Play after play after play on the screen No. 51 shed blocks to make the stop.

Finally, Donahue turned to one of his assistant coaches and asked, "Who the hell is that?"

The coach replied, "That's Don Rogers' brother, Reggie."

Donahue sat quietly for a moment, before shaking his head and saying, "That figures."

Though Reggie's play had improved, the strides he took to become a leader were of greater importance. Gone was the prince of extracurricular activity. In 1985, Reggie's roughness was deemed quite necessary as he dominated some of the best Pac-10 linemen in conference history. Rarely had anyone seen such a mixture of size, speed, and strength. Having been an outside linebacker the previous year, Reggie had received little hype considering the difficult position change. But his coaches knew very well what they had, and they didn't mind keeping their secret weapon quiet, then unleashing him on the likes of Colorado, Oklahoma State, USC, and BYU.

Following the season, despite playing on an average Washington team, Reggie was rewarded for his stellar performances with first-team All-Pac-10 Conference honors, All-West Coast honors, honorable mention All-America, and was selected by his teammates as their "Lineman of the Year." The parade of awards might have been greater still had Reggie been a known quantity at defensive tackle. As it stood to many people, though—despite his name recognition—Reggie came out of nowhere to dominate.

As soon as the season ended, Reggie was told he would be a consensus 1986 pre-season All-American, and would be a leading preseason candidate for college football's prestigious twosome: the Outland Trophy and the Lombardi Award. For the first time in his life, at least on the field, Reggie was actually Don's equal at a comparable point in their careers—something that had never happened, and something he hadn't seemed to want very much previously.

THE ALL-AMERICA TRAGEDY OF DON ROGERS

For his part, Don could not have been more proud, directing family conversations as well as interviews over to Reggie's exploits as if he himself were the proud father of a star son. The Cleveland Browns media guide prominently featured the family accomplishments, mentioning that Jackie was playing basketball at Oregon State—which by this point, she was not—but correctly notes that Reggie had played both football and basketball for UW the previous year. From *The New York Times* to *The Los Angeles Times*, almost every article that featured Don made mention of Reggie's accomplishments and expectations as well.

Due to immaturity and circumstance, Reggie's flame had extinguished on the basketball court; and, though his favorite sport, basketball was never going to be the perfect fit for an athlete of Reggie's particular talents and build. Worse for Reggie, he could not have found a bigger mismatch for his personality than highly regarded über-disciplinarian Marv Harshman.

Surprisingly, having finally attained college stardom in football didn't result in the arrogance that follows several elite athletes. At his core, Reggie was a clown—a big kid who liked to make people laugh. After all the on-court and on-field ruckuses, stardom seemed to settle him down, as though he finally understood that responsibility was part of the package. For the first time in his life, he seemed secure, stable, less easily threatened.

Or perhaps he was just too busy to act out.

Despite his prodigious basketball talent, athletically and emotionally Reggie simply was best suited to play along the defensive line, which encouraged him to go all-out on each play and make things happen—more instinct, less thinking. No longer was he restricted by an offensive system or substitution patterns. Just wind him up and let him go. The result was more than football stardom: For the first time ever, evidence existed that a composed young man, a person with discipline, manned the controls of his own immense talent.

In the spring of 1986, Reggie was elected to be a captain for his upcoming senior year—in some respects his greatest achievement.

ONE MOMENT CHANGES EVERYTHING

He'd been so many things in his young life: an understudy, a star, a disappointment, a disgruntled backup, a clown, a cheap-shot artist, a little brother, a mentor to inner-city kids, an unrealized talent, even a showoff. Reggie had the temperament and ability to lead, but like so many people, he probably needed to feel secure with himself to undertake that role. Suddenly, as a rising fifth-year senior, his peers and coaches were anointing him a captain—and the honor was due more to his character and leadership than his on-field prowess.

"Nobody on the team has competed harder this spring than Reggie. He wants to excel, and we've come to rely on him," said Washington assistant coach Jim Heacock.

Tough-as-nails head coach Don James also knew he could rely on Reggie. "He's worked harder than anyone on the team," said James. "He's become our leader."

Reggie reached out to freshmen, transfers, and new players on the team, using his knowledge of the difficulties acclimating to college life. He wanted them to feel accepted in equal standing, perhaps remembering the jeers he experienced when he first came out for the team. In awe of Reggie and the Rogers family legacy, the wide-eyed newcomers—and Reggie's peers—all viewed him as royalty.

Any athlete can attest to the social hierarchy of teams. Different rules apply to star players than to bench players. Certainly, jealousy and animosity exist, but only among players of reasonably equal talent levels who are fighting for playing time or to make the team. Safe to say, second- and third-string defensive linemen were not blaming Reggie's starting position on favoritism. He was just so clearly a superior talent that even the most self-absorbed teammates could only be glad that Reggie Rogers was on their side.

Reggie wanted to be approached by the newbies, and he valued the senior role of team social worker, utilizing the same characteristics that would someday make him a good father. Perhaps the most telling facet of Reggie's growth could be his volunteer work at the King County Department of Youth Services juvenile detention center in Seattle—where he peppered the staff with questions, intently worked with the most troubled children, signed autographs, and excitedly spoke of a career in social work after his playing days had ended.

That wasn't likely to be anytime soon. Such was Reggie's impact on the field his junior season that he was tabbed by NFL scouts as a probable first-round draft pick for the following year. And buzz abounded that, if Reggie Rogers continued to improve and had a monstrous senior season, he might actually be the very first pick in the entire draft. To say that this young man's life had completely changed would be an overstatement. If anything, after coming close to derailment, it was now back on track. Back to where it was supposed to be, just as many had always predicted.

By switching sports, Reggie had exceeded his own previous level of stardom, achieved, at least in part, by what was supposed to be, as much as what actually was. By making the All Pac-10 Freshman team in basketball, and prompting unrealized Olympic team conversations, Reggie was ascending his own personal ladder of fame. But his basketball career had hit the wall of reality well short of any really truly great accomplishment.

Even though sister Jackie was living with Loretha, and had given up sports, she was still revered around Sacramento. Why she gave it all up was never made clear, but not everyone is made for the rigors and sacrifices necessary to excel at the college level. And in the mid-'80s, with few exceptions, girls athletics were underfunded, understaffed, and lacked a passionate following. Without the ever-present support system and guardianship of her mother and brothers, it was obviously all so very different than it had been in high school. In college, achievement is realized almost exclusively by personal motivation and sacrifice. And, as Reggie had found, talent alone wouldn't suffice.

11

As the summer of 1986 commenced, the Rogers' futures were as bright, safe, and promising as any family could hope to have. Loretha was still a relatively young woman, only in her early 40s, who looked even younger still. She had born into the poverty of a segregated south, but through strong will, vigilance, luck, and discipline, she had managed to raise three singularly talented and devoted children, and they, in turn, had managed to avoid the ever-present dangers in and around Del Paso Heights.

"The boys and Jackie were always helping their mother," declared one neighbor in South Natomas, who requested to remain anonymous. "The yard was immaculate. They were a very close-knit family. To be honest, I didn't even know they were star athletes, but the two boys (Don and Reggie) were always out playing ball in the street with neighborhood kids, who would knock on their door all hours of the day."

Don was a star about to enter the final year of his initial Cleveland Browns contract, and negotiations for a long-term deal—one that would pay him as much as any safety in football—were already in the works.

Reggie himself was just months away from ascending to a commensurate level of wealth as well, possibly even more. He was already slated to appear on the cover of numerous 1986 preseason college-football publications, some predicting that he would be the top pick in the 1987 NFL draft.

Yet, one giant detour lay ahead. Out of sight, a landslide blocked the road.

ONE MOMENT CHANGES EVERYTHING

The insidious ether in America's air manifested itself in 1986. Gross materialism in our culture had found the perfect outlet for the excess of money and prosperity, leading thousands of people to scamper willingly off a figurative cliff in pursuit of a good time—or of a way to cope with the bad. Tragedies began to play out at the end of rolled dollar bills and glass pipes used to ingest cocaine. While inner cities were being blindsided by cocaine and the onset of the crack epidemic, nowhere was the drug more visibly destructive than the world of sports.

The 1986 World Champion New York Mets potential dynasty found itself single-handedly derailed by cocaine. At the time, though, with no insider knowledge or reports from behind the scenes, no one could figure out why the Mets' run ended with a single title. Doc Gooden, Darryl Strawberry, as well as others—many of the brightest young talents of the era—would never live up to their staggering potential. Some feel they were casualties of their own early success, while others believe they were simply symptoms of a greater social epidemic.

One thing, though, was closed to debate: Those young men, and many like them, were addicted to cocaine. Sure enough, several supremely talented careers never left the ground, or were ruined outright, because of a dependence on the drug.

No one knew that NFL superstar Lawrence Taylor was playing high on cocaine, or that Villanova's Denny McClain was doing lines before many of the Wildcats' games en route to the 1985 NCAA Championship. Like so many other reports and stories of lesser known athletes who disappointed or simply didn't live up to expectations before fading away, Taylor's, Gooden's, Strawberry's, and McClain's transgressions with drugs would surface gradually in news reports, arrests, stays in rehab, articles, and tell-all books as years passed.

Yet, while those downfalls were of the slow, painful kind, they weren't without precedence. There was that initial tragedy, the one that stopped the clock, the one that might have scared them straight, the shovel-to-the-face foreshadow of the calamity that was to come: The death of Len Bias.

THE ALL-AMERICA TRAGEDY OF DON ROGERS

❖ ❖ ❖

Considered one of the top classes in history, the 1986 NBA draft included Len Bias, Brad Daughtery, Roy Tarpley, William Bedford, Chris Washburn, Dennis Rodman, Mark Price, Jeff Hornacek, Dwayne "Pearl" Washington, John Salley, Ron Harper, Chuck Person, and many more.

On June 19, 1986, just two days after becoming the second-overall selection in the NBA draft, Bias celebrated in his dorm room with people who were supposed to be his friends. The entire time, he was bragging that he could snort more coke than anyone on the planet because, you see, he was invincible—or perhaps he felt he needed to be.

A few short hours later, Len Bias was dead.

Bias' overdose was front-page news across much of the world. He had Michael Jordan-level talent and charisma to match. He was about to be a Boston Celtic, the greatest team in the universe. Since Bias played his college basketball at the University of Maryland, which was in the shadow of our nation's capitol, top-flight news correspondents representing worldwide news services quickly took to the story and made it a global tragedy.

Ratcheted into warp speed by a shock that would follow just eight days later, the death, the investigation, the outcry, and the government's massive response all kept Bias' name on the front page of the *Washington Post* for the next three months. The story became Watergate in high tops, making its way into newspapers across the planet.

On the human scale, Boston Celtic star Larry Bird said Bias' death was "The saddest thing I have ever heard."

President Ronald Reagan called it "a horrible national tragedy."

At Bias' funeral, Jesse Jackson eulogized the fallen idol with the seemingly trite sentiment, "Len's in heaven dunking with the angels now."

That comment, however, is best reviewed in its unique context. Outside the occasional baseball strike, spectators had little to be cynical about in American sports. In some ways, the sports world was one big community; and fans—certainly those too who knew Bias personally—were overcome with grief reserved for the sudden, shocking loss of a beloved and admired person in the very prime of his life.

Sure, many factors came into play. That Bias was seen as a can't-miss star of the future, a player who would have given the Celtics the explosiveness and athleticism they needed to counter the Los Angeles Lakers' James Worthy, certainly contributed. Bias might well have kept the Celtics on top for many more years to come. Instead, the Celtics never won another title, while the Lakers went on to win the next two NBA championships. NBA teams are more dependent on drafts than any other sport. Any team that loses the second-overall pick without compensation suffers serious repercussions as a result.

Obviously, not everyone is a basketball fan—and not everyone lives on the East Coast. And not everyone can relate to a young man being paid millions of dollars to stuff a ball through a hoop, even if he does have a high-wattage smile. So in the end, to many, despite Bias' popularity, an undeniable truth exists within the sentiment that Bias' death was little more than a newly minted millionaire acting recklessly. That shouldn't weaken the tragedy's effect, but since many people simply couldn't relate to Bias' world, it does.

Many saw Bias' death as an once-in-a-lifetime happening, a fluke. From suburban perches and barstools several times removed, it was deemed as sad, but people did understand that those things happen from time to time.

Besides, maybe something was wrong with Bias, some inherent weakness in that superhuman frame.

Perhaps he snorted an incredible number of fat white lines.

Maybe he was an addict.

True or not, people create their own conclusions, or illusions, and then they move on. In many circumstances, that's a good thing. To survive and be happy in our world takes some denial.

THE ALL-AMERICA TRAGEDY OF DON ROGERS

So, on its own, Len Bias' death was not going to be enough to awaken America to the dangers of cocaine, not to the degree that was necessary for change. Besides, the country was in the throes of a devoted love affair with the drug, and certainly didn't want to end the relationship, which had become a symbol of the good life, of wealth and accomplishment. In 1985, well over $30 billion in cocaine was sold in the United States. Very few legal enterprises came anywhere close to achieving that figure. Besides, tens of thousands of hard-working, successful people used cocaine all the time, and almost nobody died.

Such was the perception surrounding a drug that, just four years earlier, two prominent Yale University psychiatrists—doctors who had spent years studying cocaine's effects—determined that "recreational" use was no more harmful to an individual than using alcohol or tobacco. Splashed across papers from coast to coast, their research also concluded that cocaine users did not develop a tolerance for the drug. This meant that users wouldn't become addicted because increasing amounts weren't needed to achieve the same "high" with each use.

They also concluded that death from cocaine was extremely rare.

Truthfully, it was just that—extremely rare.

However, the number of jobs lost, homes and cars repossessed, hearts literally scarred into the future, early deaths, and families shattered beyond repair were staggering—but people weren't dropping dead each day, so cocaine simply wasn't the big news it would soon become. The Yale psychiatrists completed their study with the opinion that the government's efforts, as well as the expense required to keep the drug out of the country, may be unjustified based on the actual risks cocaine posed to the public.

Still, when Don Rogers heard that Len Bias had died, he called his mother and cried. Just a week before his wedding, despite his packed schedule, Don flew to Seattle to see his brother. Instead of flying home to Sacramento, the two decided to drive the 800 miles back to Sacramento so they could spend some time together and talk about their futures.

ONE MOMENT CHANGES EVERYTHING

A week passed, and while some around the country continued to mourn Bias' death, the time had come for the Rogers family to celebrate their successes and the brilliant future that shone in their eyes.

12

Thursday, June 26, 1986—Don's wedding to Leslie Nelson was just two days away. Under a new, first-of-its-kind program set up by the Cleveland Browns, players would receive assistance to return to school and earn their college degrees; so Don was in L.A. taking his final course to fulfill his economics degree requirements at UCLA. Then Don would fly to Sacramento that evening for what promised to be a warm gathering of family and friends for his bachelor party at the downtown Hilton hotel.

Meanwhile, the Rogers home burst at the seams as relatives, friends, and teammates from all over the country arrived for the wedding. Although scheduled to be held 90 miles away in Oakland, the ceremony seemed centered at the Rogers' South Natomas home as people streamed in and out of the neighborhood all week. Over 500 guests were expected to attend the ceremony that would send Don and Leslie off as man and wife to their honeymoon in the Bahamas.

In accordance with Don's wishes, the bachelor party was going to be a sedate affair. As best man, Reggie was the organizer of the event; but how was he going to pay for it when he had so little money? Surely, it would not have felt right to ask Don. . . .

A year or so earlier, Reggie had met Terry Bolar, a black, flashy ex-athlete who would come to have a profound impact on the Rogers family and, through them, the world of sports and beyond. Before a brief stint with the New York Giants, he had played college football for Long Beach State University. After his professional career had ended, Bolar began working as an "agent's runner."

"He's one of the legends," said a Los Angeles-based sports agent back in 1987, who specifically requested not to be identified. "He showed up everywhere and talked to every kid (player). I would guess he lives in a motor home. If you have a number for him, it's probably a pay phone."

In 2007, when someone says, "agent's runner," little sophistication is required to realize what the title implies. Most sports fans, even someone with minimal knowledge of athletics, would understand that, in place of the actual agent, "runners" work to ingratiate themselves to an athlete's family. They make early and illegal contacts with potential professional athletes who are still in college, then funnel those prospective clients to their employers in exchange for a percentage of the athlete's future earnings. Terry Bolar was an agent's runner who, after his initial meeting with Reggie sometime in 1985, had embodied his role so perfectly that, by June 1986, he was calling Loretha Rogers "Mom." Bolar's employer in the summer of 1986 is uncertain, but who he began working for soon thereafter is one of several gruesome brushstrokes in a near-perfect portrait of corruption and evil.

Don's own career was safely under the care of respected lawyer and agent Steve Arnold of San Francisco, and no mention of any possible change or discontent in that relationship has ever surfaced. Yet, in the carnivorous world of sports agents desperate for their pound of an athlete's flesh, Reggie was viewed as a once-in-a-lifetime, medium-rare slice of filet mignon complete with a vintage bottle of Chateau Margaux to wash it down.

On the day of the bachelor party, when Reggie showed up at Executive Limousine to secure his brother suitable transportation from the Sacramento Airport to the Hilton, he didn't arrive alone. "Reggie obviously didn't have any money, and this guy was paying," said the manager of Executive Limousine. "He was real flashy. He was definitely from out of town. He wore a lot of gold."

The credit card receipt was signed by one Terry Bolar.

THE ALL-AMERICA TRAGEDY OF DON ROGERS

What an opportunity it must have been for the young Bolar—besides becoming Reggie's potential future representation, the bachelor party and the wedding would be a who's-who of famous NFL athletes and coaches, college stars, and various friends of Don and Reggie. Not only were many of these men potential targets, each represented possible forays into meeting or securing other famous clients as well.

Bolar must have felt as if he'd been asked to dine at Caesar's table.

First, though, they had to pick up Don. Browns' three-time All-Pro cornerback Hanford Dixon, who along with Kenny Easley and Reggie, would be in the wedding party, was the first to greet the groom as he stepped through the gate. Don was in good spirits—there were smiles all around—but he had something serious on his mind.

"He told me that he wanted me to ride with him to Oakland the next day (for the wedding rehearsal)," said Dixon. "He said he had something important to talk to me about."

The partygoers proceeded to the Hilton, where Reggie had secured a suite on the top floor. Some of the other guests, including Dixon, had also reserved rooms for the night. Between Reggie, Bolar, a few Cleveland teammates, some friends from UCLA, and some childhood friends, perhaps 25 young men were present at the Hilton that evening.

"They were a bunch of really good guys who were quiet and tipped well," said the room service waiter. "It was very laid back."

"A very mellow gathering," added the night manager of the Hilton, "[just] a couple of beers and lots of food."

Tired, Don was the first to leave the party, quietly exiting the suite to return to his family's South Natomas home to sleep. Many of the guests hadn't realized that Don had left, but no one was surprised. Never would Don want to spoil anyone's fun by drawing attention to himself in being the first to leave. Besides, there was always tomorrow, and Don's taxing schedule had taken him on a sequence of trips for business, school, and to attend to personal affairs from Cleveland to Seattle to Sacramento, then back to

ONE MOMENT CHANGES EVERYTHING

Cleveland, over to Los Angeles, and finally back to Sacramento all in a week's time.

Reggie and some of the other attendees decided to go to a nightclub located just down the street from the Hilton, but that too, was uneventful—as Thursday nights in Sacramento usually were—and the gathering broke up sometime around 2 a.m. Everyone was excited about the wedding, but also calm. The guest of honor had that effect on people. Don was always soft spoken and "in the moment," meaning that whomever he spoke to received his undivided attention.

In the hyper-masculine sports world, the word "leader" can be a treacherous and oft-challenged role. No matter what the demographic of a gathering, however—in or out of sports, be it a bunch of friends, businessmen, coaches, or community leaders—Don led quietly by example, which attracted people to him.

Don was certainly aware of his position and his authority....

Aware of his place in the lives of others.

Aware that a room full of men would gravitate toward him.

Aware of how his defensive teammates looked to him when the Browns or Bruins were backed up against their own goal lines.

Aware that the house his family lived in and the cars his family drove all originated from his talent.

So that night, an exhausted Don Rogers excused himself from the Hilton suite in exactly the same way he had moved through his entire life: with quiet dignity.

No one present that evening would have guessed that they had just seen him alive for the last time.

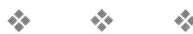

That Friday morning, the Rogers house was full of uncles and aunts, Loretha and Jackie, and, evidently, that agent's runner named Bolar. Sitting next to his mother, and probably his sister, Don ate breakfast. His appetite could not have been large. He would've spoken little.

THE ALL-AMERICA TRAGEDY OF DON ROGERS

The phone rang—Hall of Fame wide receiver Paul Warfield, the man who oversaw the dozen or so Browns players who had returned to college to earn their degrees, was on the other end. Warfield told Don who from the team's front office would be making the trip to Sacramento to attend the wedding. The two laughed because dozens of Browns were already there.

"He was great—typical Don," Warfield recalled.

One has to wonder if, just then, after hanging up, Don thought about how much his life had changed, how he had actually made it out of The Heights.

His family.

His son.

The hundreds of people in town for his wedding.

The Browns' tremendous defense.

The words from Hall of Famer Paul Warfield.

His own continued ascendancy up the ladder of NFL elite.

His place within one of the storied franchises in pro football history.

His store-bought No. 20 jerseys hanging like muumuus on the skinny kids of Sacramento, desperate to be associated with someone who had transcended their world.

These were Don's responsibilities—and he was preparing to get married, preparing to take on even more.

So in the end, the answer is probably "No." Don didn't take in a deep breath of nostalgia before heading upstairs to take a shower. Most 24-year-olds are not nostalgic. Besides, when a boy comes from the jungle, he never loses the instinct that he's being hunted.

Hunted by the competition.

Hunted by the realities inherent to his origins.

Hunted by the prejudices over the color of his skin.

Hunted by those despotic, universal laws that dictate what becomes of kids who are born into nothing.

The Rogers family had moved, but The Heights hadn't gone anywhere. Nothing had changed. The Heights were right across the street.

ONE MOMENT CHANGES EVERYTHING

Only six years removed from Norte Del Rio High School, Don was little more than a kid himself; and at times, that Browns jersey rubbing against his skin had to feel like store-bought fabric to him as well. He may have been everyone's daddy, but he wasn't ready. In the end, he only embodied the responsibilities of a 40-year-old man, but he wasn't yet a full-grown man himself.

So after hanging up with Paul Warfield, Don headed upstairs to take a shower, to catch a break from being everybody's everything. He probably hurried, scaling two stairs at a time. He probably hurried to find some relief from having everything anyone could ever want without truly knowing what to do with it all. He hurried away from everyone wanting everything from him.

At 10 a.m., a primal scream ripped the morning air, a piercing sound that others reported feeling within their houses several doors away—an agonizing release that caused the neighbors to cringe in fear. "The kind of sound you never forget," said an old man who lived next door. Thinking that an animal was being tortured, a woman two houses down knocked tables over as she frantically locked her doors. She picked up the phone, ducked behind the windowsill, and called the police.

Don was pounding on the wall of his room, and the house shook beneath the strain. He managed to cry out the words: "Ma, call for help—quick!"

Jackie dialed 9-1-1. No one remembers exactly what was said, but help was on the way.

Help is on the way.

Hang on, Don.

Let us try and save you.

Please, hang on.

Already myriad facets of the scene are too surreal, too foreign to the life of Don Rogers. Family and friends are brought to tears at the mere thought of Don calling for help. It just didn't make sense. It had always been Don to the rescue. To fathom him pleading for help was impossible.

Maybe, just maybe, out of the super-talented but fallible stars who comprised the Rogers family—perhaps the provider, the All-

THE ALL-AMERICA TRAGEDY OF DON ROGERS

American, the confidante, the hero, the groom-to-be, the 24-year-old—it was actually Don Lavert Rogers who needed help most of all.

One thing is for sure: He would never have asked for it.

Of all the people present that morning, the police report identifies Terry Bolar as the lone individual who rode with Don en route to the hospital; but that was later denied and cannot be confirmed. Why, though, was Terry Bolar even at the Rogers' house that morning? Why would he, of all people, ride with Don to the hospital? And if he didn't, why would people ever believe that he did?

Or does it matter?

For some reason, no one could stop Don from ingesting what killed him. On one hand, it seems reassuring that, no matter who rode in the ambulance with Don Rogers—a man who made life richer for everyone—someone was there, that he wasn't alone in destiny's chariot.

Yet, it's far less comforting when one realizes that his final companion might have been Terry Bolar.

13

Perhaps the human condition causes us to make involuntary assumptions about a person's success or failure. Our affection for celebrities when they please us versus our harsh judgment of them when they disappoint us exemplifies this natural tendency. Knee-jerk reactions to a person's behavior stem more from what we know about ourselves than anyone else, though; and unfortunately, even basic self-awareness is lacking in our arcane judgments. When we aren't succeeding in a way that suits us, our worst sides sometimes emerge.

So that we may better live with and accept our own imperfections—so that we may gain a modicum of control over a world that offers us no guarantees—we often react impulsively to painful situations, applying the first, easiest, or most familiar definition, one that allows us an understanding, one that allows us to move on. In this way, we each retain authority over the microcosmic worlds we found and inhabit.

Still, when a jolt of panic interrupts mundane events, it jars the memory, and time and everything within becomes a spastic blur.

To those just outside of a tragedy—media, police investigators, the inquisitive public—details are vital. They mean everything. Yet, to insiders they mean nothing. Only the tragedy matters, only the tragedy remains.

Worse still, those badly shaken souls, those most affected, are beseeched by the authorities to remember agonizing minutia regarding tiny specifics of the events leading up to their heartbreak.

ONE MOMENT CHANGES EVERYTHING

Under duress, however, all the mind really wants to do is protect itself by wandering, by forgetting.

The Rogers survivors would spend years doing everything they could to forget that fateful final Friday morning—from the moment Don awoke to the second he went downstairs to get something to eat, on to the instant that his physical being forever vanished from their lives. That day, June 27, 1986, at once changed everything and became a catalyst for changes to follow, changes that would forever alter a nation and the world of sports. Yet, atop all that change, a terrible price was exacted on a family, and the cost of that summer morning would lead to larger, even worse tragedies in future years.

Teammate Hanford Dixon would agonize over that conversation he and Don never got to have on the way to Oakland for the rehearsal dinner.

What if they actually would have had the chance to speak the previous evening?

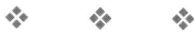

In a confusing timeline of events, some reports stated that the phone rang in Reggie's room at the Hilton; and after hearing the news, he sprang from bed and ran into the hall and began pounding on Hanford Dixon's door. He may have said, "Don's had a drug overdose," but no one's certain.

Dixon replied, "Stop messing with me."

A scramble of activity and commotion followed as Reggie and several others piled into a car and tore through the streets of Sacramento toward the Rogers' home.

Doctors at two different hospitals worked frantically on Don for six hours, unable to revive him. Though his heart had continued working off and on throughout the afternoon, blood was seeping into his lungs, denying oxygen to his brain. Attempts to revive Don halted late that Friday afternoon, when he was pronounced dead at Mercy San Juan Hospital.

THE ALL-AMERICA TRAGEDY OF DON ROGERS

Local stations in several cities interrupted programming to broadcast the news. Pending an autopsy, some hesitated to speculate about the cause, but with Len Bias' death coming just eight days earlier, a giant lump was forming nationwide in the throats of drug users and abstainers alike.

The next morning, Saturday, June 28, headlines and photos of Don appeared on the front page of every major newspaper nationwide.

No one who had ever met him could comprehend it. Sports departments argued with editorial staffs over whether main news or sports would relay the story. *The Los Angeles Times, The Cleveland Plain Dealer, The San Francisco Chronicle*, and hundreds more placed upon journalists the unenviable charge of capturing the magnitude and breadth of both Don's life and the tragedy in just a few short pages. Several writers, admitting the situation was difficult to believe, speculated uneasily that drugs were to blame.

The cause of death was not conclusive—not yet—but it didn't matter. In America, recovery is celebrity driven. As though a switch had been thrown, calls to national drug hotlines rose over 300 percent that same day, creating the first of many craters left by the meteoric impact of Don Rogers' death.

Later that day, at almost the precise moment that Don was scheduled to take Leslie Nelson as his wife—in her own father's church, no less—television stations broke with regular programming to broadcast the cause-of-death news conference from Sacramento. The Rogers family stood before the TV, staring at a smiling image of Don looking back at them from the widescreen. Upon hearing the coroner's report that cocaine had killed her son, Loretha suffered a heart attack and collapsed into Reggie's arms. Reggie lowered his mother to the sofa, and for the second time in as many days, a 9-1-1 call was placed from the Rogers' South Natomas home.

Then, with Loretha hospitalized in critical condition, Reggie was left to take control.

ONE MOMENT CHANGES EVERYTHING

❖   ❖   ❖

With a job to do, the media had assembled ten deep outside the house, surrounded still by the cars of friends and relatives, the assortment of network-logo vans, rubbernecks, and the wagons of local scribes, which seemed to stretch for miles in every direction. Mourners, family and friends—mostly black, some hysterical—came and went from the Rogers manor, and all refused or could not bring themselves to answer any questions. In the midst of tragedy, stupidity is not suspended, but magnified: Someone asked a passerby whether Don's death would rate a visit from Jesse Jackson.

But the Cleveland Browns' own Director of Security, Ted Chappelle, a tough former cop, was already on the scene. As he left the Rogers' house one afternoon after the tragedy, he whispered to reporters, "I'm worried about Reggie. He's close to having a breakdown."

No matter what the future held for Reggie Rogers—and many headlines were still to come—one cannot help but admire his courage in the days following Don's death and his mother's heart attack. By every account, when decisions had to be made, Reggie stood alone. At the time, he was 22 years old. He had no real money, no credit cards of his own. His hero and mentor had died. His mother's life was in danger. Family members were inconsolable. Hundreds of people were gathered for a wedding, and everyone in America was looking to him for several answers to one question: Why had his brother done what he did?

In what was another step in his maturity, which had been evident over the previous year, Reggie came through.

Funeral arrangements.

Interviews.

Police investigations.

His own terrible grief.

Reggie handled a perfect storm of controversy, publicity, and emotional loss—a hex that should be cast upon no human being—

and one would have to believe that somewhere, somehow, Don Rogers was proud of his little brother.

What five days before was to have been a wedding for two young people in love, was now a funeral. Everyone came, as Don would indeed warrant an appearance by Jesse Jackson, as well as more than 5,000 others. There was one terrible omission from the guest list, however: Loretha, still hospitalized, could not attend.

And what of Don's son, Little D? Only four years old as the limo pulled up to his grandmother's house to ride to the service, he saw the big shiny car and became excited. As they approached Arco Arena, he thought they were going to a Sacramento Kings' basketball game. That image offers a telling glance into the realm immediately surrounding Don's death. A full five days after the tragedy, a four-year-old boy was still unaware that his father had died. Somehow, no one had told him. Loretha was not there to do it. Reggie's hands were full. Jackie was inconsolable. Seemingly, no one had sat him down and explained what death was.

Maybe there just weren't enough steadfast hearts to do the terrible deed.

But Little D was with the Rogers' side of the family that day; and somehow, he didn't realize anything was amiss. True, he was a young child, but one can only imagine the numb masks covering the Rogers' true faces, which had to conceal not only Don's death, but perhaps the imminent demise of Loretha as well. Logically, by the time the funeral service commenced, they all had gone into survival mode, just hoping to get through the ordeal. Some of Little D's innocence would quickly be lost, however; instead of pulling up outside Arco Arena, they drove inside the building, through the bowels of the structure, and then, still in the car, they emerged near the arena floor.

Then, Little D saw his father sleeping inside the box.

The time had come to remember, to grieve.

Giant men, professional athletes with bodies made of steel, sobbed uncontrollably.

Norte's longtime basketball coach, Carl Youngstrom, sat stoically aside his wife of 40 years. Next to her were Los Angeles

ONE MOMENT CHANGES EVERYTHING

mayor Tom Bradley, and Sacramento mayor Anne Rudin. Throughout the room sat UCLA coach Terry Donahue, Cleveland Browns coach Marty Schottenheimer, Browns player representative Paul Warfield, the Grant Union School District president, NFL office reps, and some members from every NFL team, littered amongst family, friends, admirers, and several thousand others.

In a telling commentary about Don—and about the power of denial—none of the half-dozen or so speakers mentioned drugs. Then, Jesse Jackson, at a time when people still revered his close association to the late Martin Luther King and realized that he may run for president, broke the unspoken silence with a no-holds-barred eulogy that to this day is remembered as one of his finest speeches.

"Don is still teaching us profound lessons about life, even in death," Jackson said. "He is showing us the importance of how to determine our real friends. He is teaching that even the greatest among us are not perfect and that all of us are just one step away from death.

"The KKK does not kill as many black men and women as drugs do," Jackson continued. "The KKK does not come to us disguised as friends. They do not have access to our inner circles."

The crowd wept, and nodded, and prayed as Jackson, his rising voice cracking with emotion, told the mourners that God had taken Don to capture the attention of their generation.

Then he told them that God would keep taking their loved ones until they began to listen.

Somewhere in that audience—himself a major reason for those prophetic words—sat the man who provided the cocaine that killed Don.

True, no one forced Don to take the drug. Yet, between Jesse Jackson urging those in attendance to rise up and use Don's death to make the world a better place and Terry Donahue saying, "In my 15 years at UCLA, we have had some great individuals, but we have never had someone that the community loved, respected, and admired more than Don Rogers," the person who ushered Don across death's threshold sat there and somehow justified not only his role in ending a life but also his own continued existence here on earth. While that person would remain a mystery—at least for the time being—what might he have been feeling that day?

Jesse Jackson wasn't the only person offering elegant social commentary on the tragedies of that past ten days. Only a few days before Don's passing, Clark College's Robert Pritchett, coach of Reggie's best friend and Division II scoring leader, Ernest Lee, had offered eerily similar thoughts on Len Bias' death:

"I remember when I was coming up. The night before a game, some guys would be standing on the corner drinking a bottle of wine. I would try to get a sip, and a brother would say, 'You can't have none of this. You've got a game tomorrow. You've got to be at your best. You've got a future.' Twenty years ago Len Bias would not be allowed near anything that could hurt him. That guy would have said, 'No. You've been drafted by the Boston Celtics. You can't have any coke.' Today, that same guy took Bias by the hand and led him to his grave."

Over June's final two weeks in 1986, whomever or whatever "that guy" was, he suddenly seemed to be everywhere, all at once.

At funerals, assuaging one's own grief by empathizing with the unimaginably deep sorrow experienced by the deceased's immediate family is quite natural. Reggie, Jackie, and Little D sat in the front row with Don's fiancée Leslie and her family. Although he attended to Little D tenderly, Reggie mostly just stared ahead in a daze, while Jackie seemed shrunken by half as she sobbed intermittently throughout the afternoon.

After the service, the pallbearers—who included Hanford Dixon, former UCLA teammates Kenny Easley, Frank Cephous, Gene Mewborn, and Kevin Nelson (who had introduced Don to his fiancée)—gracefully loaded Don's casket into the hearse for the short ride to Chapel of the Chimes, the North Sacramento cemetery where their brother would be put to rest.

Don's Browns teammates who could not make the trip west to Sacramento, gathered in Cleveland for a memorial service that was open to the public, and which itself drew a large, somber crowd of mourners. Cleveland nose tackle Bob Golic—a graduate of Notre

ONE MOMENT CHANGES EVERYTHING

Dame, a team captain, a future broadcaster, and one of the NFL's brightest and most respected men—did his best to eulogize Don; but by his own admission, the shock and emotion of the tragedy left him unable to articulate either the collective or his personal sense of grief adequately. Unlike Jesse Jackson, who had his own photographer following him around for the Arco Arena service, no transcript of what Golic said remains.

With Don's death following Bias' by just eight days, and the national outpouring of grief, shock, and media attention, America was now eager to admit that it had a problem. Don and Bias forever became linked as symbols or, to some, victims of that problem, connected by profession, cause of death, race, era, date, celebrity, generation, and Jesse Jackson. Without pause, their deaths spawned profound changes to the laws of the country—hasty, overwrought changes that were born of good intention, panic, media frenzy, and politicians' desires to make big splashes before the upcoming November 1986 midterm elections.

As Reggie and the rest of the Rogers family were enduring a hurricane of tragedy, America was about to experience its own perfect storm of sensationalism and politics.

14

America had used cocaine for well over 100 years by 1986, which one could almost say marked an anniversary of sorts. Introduced medically here in the 1880s, cocaine was heralded as an amazing remedy for asthma, lauded as a sexual stimulant, and employed as a cure for alcoholism and morphine addiction. Still, even early on, the so-called "miracle drug" was abused. In 1891, at least 200 known American deaths occurred from overdoses of cocaine. The drug became so prevalent that, in 1906, the volume of cocaine consumed in America was equal to the amount ingested in 1975—despite only half the total population.

Perceptions began to change about 1910. Although cocaine was still widely prescribed by doctors to treat various ailments, including anxiety, Congress recognized the propensity for abuse and addiction among users and began to pass laws regulating the drug. By 1914, the Harrison Narcotics Act was passed, which made possessing cocaine illegal without a doctor's prescription. Ironically, while the Harrison Act made cocaine less available, marijuana, opium, amphetamines and other drugs, especially alcohol, boomed in popularity.

A look back at history seems to underline the assumption that human beings, inevitably and for various reasons, will find a way to alter their consciousnesses. Yet, as goes the appetites of the country, so go the laws. At one time or another in America, depending on the mood and the sensibilities of those doing the actual governing, almost all drugs, including alcohol, have been dichotomized as cure-alls or scourges, then subsequently taxed or criminalized accordingly. Despite America's insatiable thirst for varying states of consciousness, however, most alterations to our drug and alcohol policies have been enacted slowly and carefully. The agonizing lag has caught some unwary citizens in the vacuum between regulations, misinformation (such as cocaine as medicine), and legislation.

That is, until it came to "crack cocaine."

"Rock" cocaine first arose in American media in November 1984, when *The Los Angeles Times* reported that a "purer" form of cocaine, which was smoked rather than inhaled, was turning up in L.A.'s lower-income sections. *The New York Times* wouldn't publish a similar notice for nearly a year, when, on November 17, 1985, the paper ran a profile of "crack" addicts in the Bronx. Unlike coke in powdered form, which primarily had been characterized as a "wealthy" (i.e., white person's) drug that, consumed in private, was far less visible; crack was anointed with an AIDS-like panache almost immediately. Abusers weren't merely "addicted," they were "victimized" by something bigger and more powerful than themselves.

As an offshoot of poverty, crack also became a sign of bigotry. In its wake, addicts were left further impoverished, leading some—such as Maxine Waters, a U.S. Congresswoman from Los Angeles—to go so far as to promote the urban legend that crack had been introduced into America by the CIA (as AIDS was rumored to have been in the 1980s) as a method of generational genocide against minorities.

The national media, always seeking the spectacular, began to capitalize on the drug's sensational aspects: the emaciated addicts inside filthy houses, thousands of small plastic vials piled up in the hall, a crying child wandering about while his mother lays comatose in the corner. Crack was indeed tailor-made for sensationalism, drama, and blame; and before long, a single puff could enslave the strongest person for life.

Civil Rights leaders and the media demanded action against this new invader. Crack addiction, they testified or reported, was largely ignored because it was an inner-city, and therefore African-

THE ALL-AMERICA TRAGEDY OF DON ROGERS

American, affliction. Several equated the government's inertia to its apathy toward less fortunate members of our society. Though possibly true, an expensive "war" on drugs was already underway. These same activists, however, dismissed Nancy Reagan's $1 billion "Just Say No" media campaign as a quaint, lily-white approach from an out-of-touch politician who had no idea how to deal with this new, inner-city "epidemic."

Yet, "Just Say No" did have an effect. Children in schools throughout the country could recite the melodic mantra, which served to initiate conversations about drugs—an important step in preempting future abuse. "Just Say No" wasn't keeping adults with money to spare from buying powdered cocaine, though, as the estimated dollar amount of the drug sold in this country in 1986 projected to an astounding $80 billion.

Still, wealthy or middle-class cocaine abuse, rampant and destructive as it may have been, was largely an invisible problem that existed behind closed doors. Crack was different. Afforded and abused by the poor, rocks were being smoked, as well as dealt, on the street in plain sight. Violent crime involving addicts skyrocketed in these hot zones, and soon gang activity arose around the acquisition and procurement of the drug for resale. The premise was simple: An addict's appetite was so overwhelming, his urges so uncontrollable, that he would do *anything* to stay high.

Thus, the inner-city drug war couldn't be fueled by sudden altruistic bursts intended to help upper-middle class coke addicts into recovery. The battle had to be framed as "everyone's problem," the way that AIDS was being combated. Mostly seen as a homosexual disease, AIDS hadn't changed heterosexual behavior—despite the famous faces associated with the illness. Not until Magic Johnson's 1991 announcement that he was HIV-positive on national television did AIDS truly become everyone's concern. If the war on crack cocaine was going to gain momentum and public support, it needed a famous face.

In June 1986, it claimed two.

In the month following the deaths of Len Bias and Don Rogers, the three evening news broadcasts ran at least 74 segments—not simple reports, but lengthy features—profiling crack cocaine, many mentioning both young men. In the months leading up to the November elections, NBC news ran 400 separate reports on crack (15 hours of airtime). *CBS News* aired a documentary entitled *48 Hours on Crack Street*. And on September 22, 1986, *Time* decided that crack was the "Issue of the Year", while just a few weeks earlier, *Newsweek* had called crack "the biggest news story since Vietnam and Watergate." Much of the increased focus on crack, however, had resulted from a misstatement—a seemingly innocuous quote that came from Maryland's assistant medical examiner, Dennis Smyth, who said that Bias had probably died of "free-basing" (smoking crack) cocaine.

Because of this—and despite the fact that the attending physician on the day of Bias' death had announced that the drug found at the scene was regular powdered cocaine—the *Los Angeles Times*, *USA Today*, *Chicago Tribune* and *Washington Post*, among others, all elected to run Smyth's "free base" headline. Later reports that confirmed that Bias' death was the result of snorted powdered cocaine didn't emerge for almost a year, when Brian Tribble, who was accused of supplying the cocaine that killed Bias, testified in his own defense. Somehow, though, that information was buried on the back pages of the same newspapers. As for Don—due to various reporters' overzealousness and mistakes and the early confusion and ignorance as to the exact differences between crack and powdered cocaine—millions of people to this day incorrectly believe that both he and Bias died from smoking crack.

Soon thereafter, several media outlets, conflicted between fair and unbiased reporting and the presence of sensational, groundbreaking stories, were labeling crack, "America's drug of choice." It didn't seem to matter that crack wasn't even tops among cocaine users—according to one report, in 1986, 95 percent of the cocaine used in America was purchased and snorted in powdered form.

THE ALL-AMERICA TRAGEDY OF DON ROGERS

❖   ❖   ❖

The American legal system, for much of its history, was affected by a policy known as "indeterminate sentencing," which, simply put, meant that two people who commit the same crime could receive varying levels of punishment. State laws, representation, judicial philosophy—and, to some extent, race—all played a part in prison sentences.

When cocaine took the nation by storm in the 1980s, however, the country developed a punitive attitude that shifted the legal-process foundation back to a "determinate sentencing" principle that aligned punishment with set guidelines. Simply, everyone who committed a particular crime that was defined by a "determinate sentencing" mandate would receive the exact same sentence upon conviction.

Dense statistical evidence showed that mandatory minimum sentencing had not reduced drug crime in the 1960s, but public outcry against crack cocaine forced the government's hand. Congress commenced sessions to research and complete the landmark Anti-Drug Abuse Act in the fall of 1986.

Despite overwhelming evidence that neither Don nor Bias had been killed by smoking crack, the public's media-driven hysteria over the rising inner-city epidemic led the U.S. Senate's Permanent Subcommittee on Investigations to meet to discuss crack cocaine. Records from the meeting verify that the names of Len Bias and Don Rogers were cited a combined 11 times. (In later sessions to pass the Anti-Drug Abuse Act, Congress would use their names 100 times.) Politics soon took hold in what would be the opening salvo of a coming frenzy—a veritable hangman's posse of elected leaders determined to pass harsh, groundbreaking drug-sentencing guidelines into law in time for November midterm elections. To do this in such a short span of time would require circumventing typical protocol, not to mention a Congressional urgency never before chronicled in legislative history. Nevertheless, the media and much of the American public would see their wishes granted, as an overreaching drug bill was rushed to the floor—one that called for billions in new spending and mandatory federal prison sentences for relatively small quantities of crack. Possession of five grams of crack would now warrant a five-year prison sentence, the same penalty for possessing 500 grams of powder cocaine.

At the time, crack cocaine had been on the streets of America for just over two years. So, were members of Congress even fully aware of what they were voting on?

On September 26, 1986, Senator Charles Mathias of Maryland admitted, "Very candidly, none of us has had an adequate opportunity to study this enormous package. It did not emerge from the crucible of the committee process."

Representative Trent Lott of Mississippi appeared to agree when he stated, "In our haste to patch together a drug bill—any drug bill—before [Congress adjourns], we have run the risk of ending up with a patchwork quilt that may not fit together into a comprehensible whole."

So whispers of levelheaded restraint were emitted, but perhaps too few, too quietly. The media was demanding immediate and major action, though; and politicians could not risk campaigning against the bill's proponents after taking a "soft stance" on the national security issue of the day—the "biggest story since Vietnam and Watergate," no less.

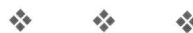

In 1986, alcohol was the primary factor in roughly half the nation's traffic fatalities. Alcohol also contributed or directly caused 100,000 deaths in America that year; but with its lobbies paying millions to elect sympathetic politicians, no Congressman ever campaigned to have alcohol criminalized.

During the 1986 Congressional hearings on cocaine, at least seven college students died from binge drinking alcohol. Alcohol was legal, however, and served as an official sponsor of professional and college sports; so those seven students faded into history, and with the exception of their families, their names have been forgotten.

THE ALL-AMERICA TRAGEDY OF DON ROGERS

Because the 1986 Anti-Drug Abuse Act was rushed into law, it left behind a startlingly thin legislative record. Rather than volumes of notes and information one might expect from exhaustive studies and arguments carefully considering all sides, comparably few records exist, though the repercussions of the 1986 Anti-Drug Act are still very much in evidence today.

Although the Act aimed to rid the legal system of economic and racial bias—as far as cocaine was concerned—the exact opposite effect was often achieved. Arresting people and throwing them in jail became paramount to the "War on Drugs." Yet, unlike crack dealers—many of whom were selling on inner-city streets in plain sight—cocaine dealers were more often working with mid-level dealers in private residences. Expensive, time-consuming sting operations, along with informants, were required to bring those dealers down. Because those processes were painstakingly difficult, a motivated and keen-eyed street cop could make more crack arrests in a single day than a multimillion-dollar sting operation could make in a year.

Though many in Congress admitted that they barely understood the repercussions of their votes, on October 27, 1986, the Anti-Drug Abuse Act became federal law. In nine years, the federal prison population would double in size.

Amidst much protest from those advocating rehabilitation over imprisonment, the lawmakers finally received the numbers they hoped to create: Cocaine use in America decreased for the first time in 16 years, dropping a reported 30 percent over the following 12 months.

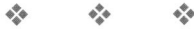

Even by 1986, officials had debated drug testing college athletes for years. In their first step toward year-round testing—what was considered an experiment—the NCAA had decided in January to begin testing athletes at championship events. The mandate was handed down six months before Len Bias or Don had died.

ONE MOMENT CHANGES EVERYTHING

Though some schools, such as Penn State, did test their athletes for recreational drug use on occasion, most did not.

Civil libertarians wondered: Why test athletes for drugs when public safety is not involved? Others worried that, if you begin to test college students, where will it end? Mercury Morris—a onetime star running back on the great 1970s Miami Dolphins Super Bowl Champions who recently had been released from prison after serving a three-year sentence for cocaine distribution—told *Time* magazine: "I would worry more about a surgeon on cocaine than an athlete."

Directly resulting from the media attention surrounding Rogers and Bias, the NCAA now gained the necessary groundswell of support and unilaterally began testing its athletes for drugs in 1987. In 2007, with steroids and other performance enhancers, drug testing, a common practice, seems logical—we've come to accept it without much debate. As of 1987, however, widespread testing had never been done and was met with hand-wringing protest. The argument against testing was that bus drivers, cops and pilots—people who held our lives in their hands—certainly needed to be clear-headed, above the throes of addiction. Public safety and accountability is the most important component of their jobs.

Of course, we had to protect the children, and after Bias and Don died that summer, the perceived urgency to do something about this "epidemic of death" was accepted as an irrefutable point of national security.

But by testing college students, was the NCAA really looking out for the public? Or was it protecting its multibillion-dollar industry? Was sports participation a privilege that obliges the athlete to live responsibly and maintain a clean existence? Or were sports voluntary extracurricular activities wherein drug testing became another example of Big Brother gaining more ground on our private lives?

The issues were complicated and remain so today. Yet, that didn't keep the NFL from jumping aboard. After all, the league had even more to gain from the well being of its athletes, not to mention protecting its reputation as a form of "family entertainment." Sam Wyche, then head coach of the Cincinnati Bengals, rang the alarm when he said, "We've got to do something. People are dying around us."

The 1982 NFL collective bargaining agreement called for one drug test per year per player, and had yet to expire. Despite protests and challenges from the players' union, after the death of Don Rogers, Commissioner Pete Rozelle and the NFL announced that year-round drug testing would commence with the 1987 season.

Within days of Don's death, more than 15 Seattle-area reporters contacted University of Washington Athletic Director Mike Lude, each inquiring about the university's drug-prevention mechanisms. In the aftermath, the public demanded to know what the University of Washington was planning to do to keep its athletes safe.

"The two deaths have turned loose, for lack of a better cliché, an emotional Mount St. Helens," said Lude. "If someone focuses on athletics as the cause of the problem, that's unfair."

Lude went on to say that he thought the public was overreacting, but he was in the minority. Emotionally, the country was incensed.

15

Though Loretha gradually regained her health following the heart attack, every mother loses part of herself when a child dies. She was only 43, leading some to surmise that Don—who, even though further tests revealed nothing, did experience an abnormal heart-stress test at UCLA—may have died from a genetic defect that was magnified by stress and cocaine. However, that thesis never was explored thoroughly.

To those who knew her, Loretha had lost a vitality that she would never regain. Later interviews with her reveal a deeply pained woman who refused to believe that drugs killed her son. Reporters would subtly refer to her slurring speech, and, while alcohol would play a role in her future, the slurring was more likely the result of depression—a sickness that runs in the Rogers family—or her heart medication.

Don's grave is located at Chapel of the Chimes in the northernmost quadrant of Del Paso Heights, just a few short miles from the Rogers' home. The cemetery is in a quiet, windswept area, wide open and flat, that had once been both farmland and a horse-grazing pasture. Even today, it is not yet encircled by development. The grounds themselves are immaculately maintained and still uncrowded.

When she felt strong enough to move about, Loretha started spending long hours at Don's grave, talking and praying with her son.

"Even in the dark, when I'm alone there," she said. "I know Don is there. And I know he won't let anything happen to me."

ONE MOMENT CHANGES EVERYTHING

Perhaps sensing her own pending mortality, Loretha announced to the family that she had purchased the plot next to Don for herself.

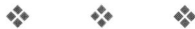

After Don's death, all eyes turned toward Reggie as the de facto head of the Rogers family. In the days following the tragedies, his impressive leadership and fortitude withstood an overwhelming tsunami of adversity that would've swept weaker men away. Washington teammate tight end Rod Jones believed that, contrary to Browns director of security Ted Chappelle's assessment, Reggie was actually holding up well.

"When the accident happened, I guess everyone fell apart," Jones told the *Seattle Post-Intelligencer* on July 2. "Now Reggie is pulling the family together. He's taking care of business and wants friends around."

Concerning how Don had died, Jones emphatically agreed with everyone else who knew Don, when he said, "I don't believe Don would do that to himself—he's not that kind of person."

But the facts were the facts. If nothing else, outwardly Reggie was keeping himself and his brokenhearted family together. For that alone, he faced the trauma as well as anyone could expect. But sometimes time has to pass before the aftereffects of tragedy bubble to the surface, and their impact on an individual can be varied and devastating.

Unfortunately, such would be the case for Reggie Rogers, who, a month after Don's death, returned to Washington to begin preseason practice for his senior year. Teammates understood that he very much wanted to bury himself in activity to avoid reflection. He just wanted to play. In fact, Reggie had told his mother that he was mostly worried about what would happen when the season ended.

"Not having anything to do but think," she'd said, "worried him a great deal."

THE ALL-AMERICA TRAGEDY OF DON ROGERS

Since 1971, his first season as head coach at Kent State, Don James had made a habit of meeting with his team's seniors to set goals and establish expectations. Another facet of those meetings was to warn his players about the dangers of drugs and alcohol. Apparently, James was taken aback by Reggie's reaction when he explained that even the casual use of alcohol could result in serious problems.

According to James, Reggie asked, "What basically is the problem with social drinking?"

"I told him that it was a drug—a chemical dependency," said James. "Then I commented about battered women and neglected children, a lot of them suffering from alcohol abuse. We talked about the dangers of driving under the influence."

Reggie clearly understood the dangers of drugs and alcohol better than most. His father had been arrested twice in 1984 for drunk driving and would again be arrested soon after Don's death. Reggie may have flirted with experimentation during adolescence, but all testimony from coaches and friends indicates that Reggie religiously abstained from drugs. Though the same was believed of his brother, Reggie wasn't one bit interested in illegal substances.

But Reggie did like to have a drink now and then, and he told Coach James as much. He didn't see the problem, especially since it was legal. Most Washington coaches and players would have agreed with him. James kept after Reggie, trying to get him to understand, but to no avail. Whether James knew of Reggie's father's problems with alcohol is unclear—perhaps he keenly sensed that Reggie's makeup was more "sensitive" to inebriants than most people. That a coach was looking out for his team's leader, a great player who had lost his only brother a month earlier, was far more likely.

"A lot of us will never have to go through that kind of adversity, " said James. "You never know how anyone's going to react to something like that, especially at such a young age."

Truthfully, Reggie's belief that alcohol was in no way harmful would've meant far less had the future unfolded without further tragedy, which, unfortunately, would not be the case.

ONE MOMENT CHANGES EVERYTHING

Besides the grief that clung to him at all times—a grief that Reggie's teammates couldn't help but notice had transformed their team's captain into something of a subdued loner—Reggie also had to contend with the media. Reggie and Don were public figures, and the public wanted to know how Reggie was dealing with his brother's death. As a preseason All-American, Reggie was slated for a big senior season, and media nationwide besieged Washington with requests to interview the team's star defensive tackle.

Of course, concerning sports, publicity translates to revenue, so most of those requests were granted. But how Don died was far more important than the fact that he died or that Reggie was still mourning that loss. In short, reporters oftentimes were blatantly insensitive, asking barbed questions of a young man whose brother had died but who had done nothing wrong himself. In 2007, no sports information director would tolerate the same litany of questions hurled forth by those journalists:

"Did Reggie ever use drugs?"

"Did Reggie use drugs with Don?"

"Was Reggie with Don when he did the cocaine?"

Given their close relationship, many people assumed that Reggie must've been using as well. Any SID who would allow an amateur athlete to face the same interrogation would've been fired the next day.

"That was my brother, not me...."

"I'm not Don...."

The scenario, Reggie's responses, would've been unfathomable just a few months earlier. The answers were painful reactions to invasive questions aimed to probe at Reggie's fraternal love. While some may feel the media was well within its right to ask any question it deemed pertinent, had Don died of murder, of suicide, while hang gliding, those same reporters would not have been so empowered. Rather, they dissected Reggie's personal, private pain in public view.

But such is the fine line of the public's right to know....

But in saying, "I'm not Don," Reggie found himself forced to distance himself from his best friend and hero—someone he loved more than anyone on earth. In all likelihood, he was still unable to accept that Don was gone. He was just 22 years old.

❖ ❖ ❖

As the college football season was set to begin, Congressional hearings kept Don in the news while legislators invoked his name on an almost daily basis. Instead of lessening, the media circus surrounding Reggie actually intensified. He couldn't escape it.

Sensing that the media had built a damaging headline around him—by associating him with his brother's cause of death rather than Don, the man—Reggie announced that, in order to clear his name once and for all, he would volunteer for a drug test to be administered by the university. That Reggie suddenly cared about his reputation (or his draft status), the bizarre change in character reeked of an illicit sports agent's micromanagement, even if made with the best intentions. The ACLU, however, would not let that happen.

In 2007, such a move seems calculated; but Reggie, anxious to lift the veil of suspicion and alleviate the pressures heaped upon him by association—albeit a blood association—hired a private firm to have himself tested for drugs.

Standing at a distance, this particular moment in the Rogers' history is poignantly unique. Consider Reggie at this point: A 22-year-old man with a history of emotional fragility thrust into the focus of an unwarranted media witch hunt. For him to suggest such a contemporary solution to deflect the negative that threatened to swallow him whole was a stroke of inspired, but desperate brilliance.

As drug users continued to be demonized by a bloodthirsty national media, libertarians saw their greatest fear realized in the form of college drug testing: Citizens were being considered guilty until otherwise proven innocent. All the while, proponents offered their own polarization: "What does anyone who isn't on drugs have to fear from drug testing?"

Lost in all this was the fact that Reggie Rogers was supposed to be having fun. This was his senior season of college football, his last year of college. Only a few years earlier, both of these milestones escaped guarantee; but what should have been a time for celebration became a time for survival, for moving forward, for moving on.

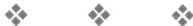

Around Seattle, Reggie remained a king-sized star in a city chock full of rabid Husky supporters. Washington sold out most of its games years in advance, and Reggie was asked to sign dozens of autographs wherever he went. His picture was plastered on billboards to promote the upcoming season, placed on the cover of game programs, and even adorned the glossy fronts of game tickets. The exposure his image and name recognition was getting was all that a forward-thinking college athlete hoping for an NFL career could ever hope to receive.

Fame: The once-per-month meal that never tastes as good as it looked in the picture.

NFL contract: The carrot waved before a college athlete's nose between those meals.

Visibility is a two-way street. On one hand, college athletes can become poster children for the NCAA, elevating their marketability and even opinions about their abilities, simply by following instructions. On the other hand, their actions are now representative of an entire institution—their school—and their mistakes can become national news. If that negative visibility arises, athletes can expect the school to protect their privacy as much as possible, but what if they didn't make any mistakes at all?

Reggie had done nothing wrong, but at some point, university officials felt that he was strong enough to be thrown beneath network buses as one after another rolled over him. It's only natural to hope that a bit of sensitivity accompanied those hit-and-runs.

THE ALL-AMERICA TRAGEDY OF DON ROGERS

The 1986 Washington football media guide is a completely different story. Reggie was presented as the player the coaching staff had anointed as the face of Huskies football—one of the most storied and tradition-rich programs in the country. Just three pages in is a full-page game photo of Reggie, the sort of "glamorous" publicity shot that any athlete would frame and keep forever.

When one comes to Reggie's player profile, however, the hard reality returns. His otherwise glowing bio begins, "Older brother, Don, former outstanding safety at UCLA and a starter for the Cleveland Browns, died tragically last summer. . . ."

One would hope that the season's onset would've provided better shelter from the storm. Several "Reggie Carries the Torch for his Family" articles did appear in various papers nationwide, so obviously some journalists were pulling for him to persevere and thrive. Yet, in retrospect, perhaps the school's publicity department could've protected him better. Reggie was in a position to bring glory to Washington—so why, unnecessarily, would they continue to saddle him with tragic reminders as news and reports of the event were saturating the media ad nauseam? Maybe the opening sentence was an attempt to enlighten those few people who were somehow still ignorant of Don's death. Maybe the school intended to preempt people from asking Reggie the same tired questions.

Both explanations seem unlikely—if anything, mentioning Don encouraged even more inquiries on the topic. In contrast, the player whose profile immediately preceded Reggie's in the media guide apparently enjoyed rafting, fishing, and playing softball. The player listed directly after Reggie is one of three children, and he liked working with ceramics. Quaint, mildly interesting tidbits remind the reader that these are only young men, who are, after all, merely amateurs. Someone reading the guide may not remember those nuggets, but he knows that a player likes working with ceramics because the media guide says so.

What would people remember after reading about Reggie?

That he had registered 15 tackles for loss in his first year playing a new position?

ONE MOMENT CHANGES EVERYTHING

That he managed the transition from basketball to football with his brother's guidance?

That his stellar performance in the 1984 NCAA Tournament upset Mike Krzyzewski's Duke squad, earning Washington a trip to the Sweet Sixteen?

Not likely.

Media guides serve as the bibles of beat reporters, sports journalists, NFL scouts, opposing coaches, boosters, and fans alike. They're sent to newspapers and alumni throughout the country. Since Reggie was a preseason All-American, the star of what promised to be a very good Huskies squad, his profile would be referenced thousands of times throughout the unfolding season. With every spectacular play, with every camera close-up, everyone would be reminded unnecessarily that Don's death was the preeminent fact in Reggie's career.

Just as renown had graced Reggie based on his own achievements, without compromise or caveat, he was cast once again into Don's shadow. Though he would soon emerge to claim his own place in the spotlight, chance and momentum were conspiring against him.

And Don was no longer there to warn him.

16

With the NFL season about to begin, public response to Don's death remained volatile and sharply divided—and everyone wanted a say. Outside of the hard-bitten world of sports, and locally in Cleveland, many people responded to Don's death with a sympathetic outpour.

Highly regarded UC-Berkeley sociologist Harry Edwards, then a consultant for the San Francisco 49ers, claimed in a 1986 *Time* magazine article that we are living in a "high" society: "The inescapable image emerges of a nation consumed in drug taking, both legal and illicit. The fact that we have by tradition placed our athletes upon a pedestal does not elevate them above prevailing cultural tides."

Still, in the end, the rush to find answers to "why" stars use drugs results in nothing definitive. A little truth is present in all theories, but one common factor seems to indicate a simple truth: Fame and stardom won't bring happiness, but that doesn't sway Americans from desperately craving prominence.

When, from a distance, people experience tragedies comparable to Don Rogers' overdose—suicide, recklessness, carelessness—a death by sin or excess shortens the figurative leash on their emotive response. Oftentimes, when confronted by the stark truth, people respond angrily to what they deem as an act of betrayal.

Still, some Cleveland football fans refuse to see Don's death in any colors but the unforgiving black and white. They don't care what kind of pressure Don was under—to them, he was a rich, spoiled athlete who, by choosing to use cocaine, stole from "their" team a vital component of success. From this perspective, because Don's actions deprived them of their refracted glory, his death is seen as the ultimate act of selfishness. They put their faith in Don, and he failed them. Others may see Don's death as just another unfortunate result of what it means to grow up in poverty, or what it means to get so much so quickly without being prepared to deal with it. Answers vary, but no one can deny the startlingly high level of reaction to Don's death.

On the 20th anniversary of his passing, in 2006, a longtime staff member at *The Cleveland Plain Dealer* reported that the newspaper received more letters in response to Don's death than any other news story in its 150-year history—an increase that, at the time, was estimated to be three-fold over anything before or since. That Browns fans responded in droves with such passion comes as no surprise. For years, they've been known as the most loyal fans in the NFL. Despite an overall record that is well below .500, 99 percent of the seats are filled at Browns home games despite some of the most extreme weather in football.

Those letters spanned the breadth of reasoning, of emotions, of the highs and lows of literacy. People who weren't accustomed to expressing themselves in writing were inspired to take the time to send in their thoughts. Touching, vicious, caring, racist, insightful, overreaching, some of the letters were genuinely brokenhearted while others emanated disappointment over a wasted opportunity that the writers claimed they themselves would never squander. Still, even they would refer to No. 20 as "Don" or even "Donnie," as his friends and coaches would sometimes call him. As of 1986, many avid fans were viewing players as their friends or possessions, a sort of live-action fantasy league before such pastimes existed; but "tough love" may best describe even the most poignant rejoinders.

"I cannot forgive Don ..." began one letter.

"Wasn't our cheering him enough?" asked another.

One more ended with, "Who is going to play safety for us now?"

For those in Cleveland who actually did know Don—those who worked with him, who won and lost games with him—they

THE ALL-AMERICA TRAGEDY OF DON ROGERS

now faced the unenviable position of a future without their teammate and coworker. They somehow had to navigate a politically correct trinity that was at once part homage, part condemnation, and part indignation, while struggling to rise above the public's thinly veiled suspicion that most professional athletes—specifically African-American stars—were getting high on drugs.

Under owner Art Modell, the 1986 Cleveland Browns were a family-run business unlike any modern conglomerates common to professional sports today. The team was run in a hands-on manner typical of the medium-sized business models of the era, and the Browns' staff and employees handled everything and knew everyone, including the players' families. To keep costs down, the team's training camp was held at nearby Lakeland Community College; and many of the players spent their entire careers in a Cleveland uniform. The franchise had a symbiotic relationship with city and employees alike—they were a *family*, which made Don's death twice as complicated, affecting every remote corner of the organization.

Drug use had become a hot-button issue in a volatile America, so no one from inside or outside the franchise would be allowed to forget that Don died doing something illegal. Coupled with the country's newest, ultra-funded war on drugs and Don's status as a role model for children, teammates and staff found themselves in the delicate position of relegating their sadness. Presenting a public face that insisted drugs run counter to organizational philosophies became paramount, as was the policy that those who use drugs should be condemned.

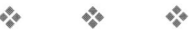

Though some fans remained unforgiving, the Browns refused to brush Don aside. Game programs feature tributes, and the 1986 Cleveland media guide opened with a commemorative photograph of No. 20. Wearing a dark home jersey, Don is seen thrusting his right fist above his head, cheering after the defense held on third down. Nothing like the high-resolution photos found on today's

ONE MOMENT CHANGES EVERYTHING

websites, Don's picture is black and white and a bit grainy. Perhaps it was raining when the photo was taken—the background is blurry, and only Don is in focus. In short, the photo is very Browns-like. A gritty, "any-era" shot from a team and franchise that never seems to change or modernize—much to the delight of its incredibly loyal fan base.

Even compared to the photogenic Bruin Blue uniforms that Don wore in college, that black-and-white image is one of his best remaining photos. The shot reflects the juxtaposition of exaltation and control. Don's manner, despite the exaltation, is well short of frenzied; and it almost looks as if he's shielding his face from the sun as he walks into the wind.

That was the real Don Rogers—celebrating and holding back, spent and victorious, always seeing more work to be done. He doesn't jump about or dance or taunt. He can't let down.

Only about one in every 12,000 high school athletes ever goes on to sign a professional contract, and far fewer actually ever make a professional roster. So when a player accomplishes what Don had—UCLA All-American, Rose Bowl MVP, college all-star games, NFL playoffs—thousands of photographs are left behind. Of course, many out-of-focus shots never leave the high school or *Sports Illustrated* darkroom, so almost every available image of Don is vibrant; and many, particularly some of his Rose Bowl photos, are spectacular.

Yet, of all the images that remain—shots focusing on the whites of his eyes searching for a target, photos of him preparing to separate receiver from the ball or from their senses—instead of heroism, the media-guide picture of Don deftly manages to convey burden, struggle, restraint, and loneliness. One can sense that, due to his recent death, the media-guide photograph was placed with the purpose of showing that a man worth knowing was now gone.

At the same time, the image may lead to the realization that no one really knew Don Rogers—especially when his closest friends and family were genuinely blindsided by the cause of his death.

So the lingering question of "Why?" may be simply unanswerable. Speculation can't separate the disappointment of those who knew Don, who cheered for Don. When they see that photo, the resignation of never knowing "why" probably reminds them that they'll never be able to understand.

He appears so completely self-contained in the photo, which he seemed to be in life as well. He didn't complain. He didn't drop excuses for his failures. He didn't give anyone any indication what walking a mile in his shoes might have been like. He gave no clues.

A photo can't answer the most complex questions, but maybe it can give a sense of closure instead of ever more mystery. One answer is clear though: We are forced to surmise what people will think and say about us after we are gone.

Beneath the picture is a quote from Rogers' star teammate, nose tackle Bob Golic: "I liked watching Don practice and play in games. His style was inspirational. As friends and teammates, we have to remember with gratitude the things Donnie gave us."

…The things Donnie gave us.

Only weeks after his death, amidst a shocked and angry country dealing with the deaths of two men most could only fantasize of becoming, Bob Golic's comments cut to the core. He was probably speaking about the team when he wrote "us," but actually he subtly reminded the fan base and the media that there was much more to Don Rogers than how he died. Surely, Golic was chosen to pen those words because he was considered beyond reproach during America's witch-hunt for drug-using athletes. Golic wasn't telling people they had to love Don or that they should overlook his faults—it was far too soon for that, and Cleveland fandom, not to mention America, was still too raw—but he did gently ask everyone to step back and appreciate something about the man, because that's what he intended to do.

After all, Don was *only* a football player—a humble and talented, but flawed 24-year-old man whose death already had mobilized massive changes to our federal drug-sentencing laws and altered the country's perception of the necessity and legality of drug testing. Yet the impact and repercussions stemming from his death were just beginning. His overdose was about to catalyze other unforeseen and far-reaching changes to people's lives both in and out of the realm of sports.

In reviewing his sentiment, Golic's understated approach was understandable (and could've been mandated by the team). A war was underway; and in 1986, football was the cleanest of entertainment marketed directly to entire families. Cheerleaders may have had their days, but Janet Jackson halftime wardrobe malfunctions did not exist. Tattoos were still for sailors. Rap music and culture, outside of the inner cities, was relatively unheard of. For the most part, the public's perception of players' off-field activities mirrored their own: dull and unremarkable as a Christmas ham. In what he was saying, Golic embarked on new territory. The phrase "self-medicating" had yet to enter our collective consciousness. Drugs were the enemy; and, by praising a friend of the "enemy" too enthusiastically, in many circles his comments would have spurred certain disgust and eye rolling. While Don's community service no doubt softened some negative reaction in a time that many sportscasters would express little to no empathy for someone who died snorting cocaine, Golic uttered the first reasonable whisper reminding people that Don was a human being, a friend, and a fabulous football player who, off the field, never hurt a soul.

The Browns players and coaches loved Don, just like his family, friends, neighbors, the beat reporters, and the competition. Just about anyone who had met him or who knew him had the utmost respect for him. In the years since his death, as the era's confusion dissipated, the positive sentiments have only grown. Echoing the thoughts of those very same souls, Terry Donahue remarked, on the 20th anniversary of Don's death: "I miss Donnie. Not knowing him later in life, it's such a shame. . . . I was so fond of him."

In the immediate aftermath of Don's passing, however, smaller concerns demanded attention. The media guide had to be pulled from the printers and altered to account for the tragedy. On the field, Marty Schottenheimer had to reconfigure his team to account for losing Don, who had been the centerpiece of a young, vicious, and dominating defense. The Browns would know great success in the post-Rogers years, but his death was still the most devastating loss the franchise could've endured. Len Bias' demise ended the Celtics dynasty—a team for which he never played—and prompted the resignations of Maryland's basketball coach and athletic director. Don's absence kept the talented Browns from making it to the Super Bowl.

In 1986 and 1987, Cleveland would advance to the AFC Championship game each year to face the Denver Broncos only to lose by a combined eight points. Heading into 1986, after being voted All-Conference the previous year, the NFL consensus was that, entering his third season, Don had become one of the league's top three safeties and could embody that mantle for some years to come. Of course, injuries and tragedies happen; but had Don not succumbed to cocaine on June 27, 1986, he would have been the starting safety in each contest.

Had Don been there, the Browns might well have won.

The 1986 AFC Championship was the year of "The Drive," courtesy of John Elway. Facing a vicious win, a seven-point deficit, and 98 yards to go with only five minutes remaining, Elway led the Denver stampede over the Browns and 80,000 of their maniac loyalists to score the tying touchdown. Unable to recover with just 30 seconds left, the Browns eventually lost the game when the Broncos' Rich Karlis hit a field goal in overtime. "The Drive" elevated Elway to icon status; but what if his defensive counterpart, Don Rogers, was on the field in that 1986 AFC Championship game? Would "The Drive" have even occurred?

Though some, especially in Denver, would consider such a theory sacrilegious, Elway did complete several passes in the middle of the field—and several were literally inches beyond the reach of safety Chris Rockins, Don's replacement. Although a fine player, Rockins was never going to make anyone forget Don Rogers, who had played against Elway in college and knew some of the quarterback's tendencies.

ONE MOMENT CHANGES EVERYTHING

"I've always thought that, maybe, one Donnie play—a hit or interception—would have put us over the top and got us into the Super Bowl," said Hanford Dixon. "He was that kind of a player."

17

Just as his senior year was about to begin, Reggie was forced to undertake the horrible task of flying to Cleveland to clean out his brother's apartment. No one else would. Like all the burdens, which some call responsibilities, that had been piled on his shoulders since Don's death, Reggie handled this charge stoically, though later he would refer to that weekend as his toughest yet.

Facing those burdens began to wear him down, and Reggie started telling friends and family that he was considering giving up football—the one, final respite he had from all the pain. Quitting wasn't an option, though. People expected big things from him. Moreover, people relied on him. Though he'd lived a dozen lifetimes since insisting that he belonged on that JV team, where life was easier, he bucked up once again and pushed forward.

After the voluntary drug tests had proven he was clean, he realized there was little more he could do or say or answer to anyone. Limiting his interviews, he politely began to steer questions toward his goals for the season and the Huskies' goals for the year, for which they'd open ranked No. 15 in the nation. If pushed by an unpleasant reporter, he would politely repeat the worn mantras again and again and again:

"That was my brother. . . ."

"I'd rather not talk about it. . . ."

Reggie dedicated his senior season to Don.

Everyone, from the press to teammates and coaches, was impressed by Reggie's fortitude as he continued to face profound adversity. His work ethic in practice and his stellar performance in training camp were exactly what teammates and coaches had come to expect. Yet, that same level of play lessened any concern others might have felt for him. Besides, like Don, Reggie never asked for special treatment. Despite all the on-field cheap shots and dust ups, off the field he'd always been a big teddy bear, slow to anger. He just wanted to be left alone to play football—or survive. In fact, football equaled survival. Not only was the game one of few constructive escapes Reggie still had, it was the only way he could save his family as well.

Although some people saw the cause of Don's death as reprehensible, to friends, family, and especially Reggie—now that his brother was gone—the sudden nature of the loss was surpassed by its magnitude. "Void" didn't cover the feeling.

Reggie probably realized that he'd never come close to replacing his brother, but he did possess the same golden ticket. If he could only follow through, he could save everyone, make Don proud, and, by going pro, replace much of what had been taken away.

Don was in the final year of his very first NFL contract. Although mere pocket change by today's standards perhaps, that contract had elevated his entire family from poverty.

But then there were taxes.

And then his agent took his percentage.

And then Don purchased a new home, not to mention several cars, for his family.

And then he got an apartment in Cleveland.

And then he had to make sure that Little D was set up well.

And then he had a huge wedding and honeymoon to finance.

So a modest nest egg may have been left over, but it couldn't have been much. The real money was going to come with the new contract that would coincide with a fourth season that Don never reached. To make matters worse, the insurance company that handled all the Browns was fighting tooth and nail to avoid paying the family any money at all. Loretha's health was deteriorating; and those close to the family assert that Don's death had the most intense impact upon Jackie, whose sadness seemed to know no bounds. And she had no idea what to do with her once-promising life.

In every sense, Reggie was stranded on an island that few others, let alone 22-year-olds, could imagine. How could anyone understand—not only his personal pain—the intense pressure that he was under to perform and react?

Nevertheless, Reggie set forth on a mission, just not one he chose to embrace.

The Washington Huskies schedule opened in Seattle against Cris Carter, Chris Spielman, and the No. 10 Ohio State Buckeyes powerhouse. Though OSU was heavily favored, the Huskies had surprisingly little trouble. The Buckeyes double- and triple-teamed the 6-foot-6, 280-pound Reggie all game, allowing the rest of the Purple Reign defense to dominate in a 40-7 drubbing.

Reggie played well, and, on national television, the opposing coaches sang his praises.

"One game down, 11 to go. Just got to keep my mind occupied, stay focused, and maybe things will be okay," he may have thought.

Washington media guide in hand, the game's commentators and radio announcers kept reminding viewers of Don's death just eight weeks earlier; and with Columbus, Ohio, being just 125 miles from Cleveland, the country's attention was diverted from Reggie's outstanding performance. People may have been sympathetic, but he was under an oppressive microscope.

Still, Reggie had played like the All-American that he was supposed to be. He led the team in every possible category, and it had gotten so opponents rarely even tried to run in his direction.

During the four-week break before Washington played Alabama in the Sun Bowl, in the hope of keeping his family together, Reggie returned home to Sacramento, only to find that things were not going well.

ONE MOMENT CHANGES EVERYTHING

❖ ❖ ❖

Money was tight. Jackie was at loose ends. Loretha was struggling with Don's death, too—and continued visits to his grave, where she prayed, which, while helpful, only numbed part of the pain.

"Whatever happened to him didn't happen in my house. I'm still not at peace with myself over Donald," she told the *Sacramento Bee*. "Some mornings, I wake up crying. Some nights, I go to sleep crying. I don't understand it. I do a lot of praying. They say God may not come when you want him to, but he's right on time."

Late one October night, a car had run up onto the sidewalk and crashed into a chain-link fence at—of all places—Grant Union High School. When the police arrived, they had found that Loretha was driving, and worse, that Little D was inside the car. They had no choice but to arrest her and charge her with driving under the influence and child endangerment. The heartache was bearing down on her.

In just a few months, so long as he stayed healthy, Reggie would be earning enough money to support his family for the rest of their lives—just not yet. That potential didn't help them make their house payments or fend off creditors. Don's money was in limbo; perhaps it was spent, perhaps it had just disappeared. Nothing was coming in, though, and the black cloud included gawkers driving past the Rogers' home day and night for a glimpse at darkness.

Down time was difficult for Reggie, period. Being in the house that Don built wasn't helping either. To soothe himself in his off hours, Reggie took to drinking beer. Men hung out doing the very same thing on half the porches in Del Paso Heights—so why shouldn't he? But Reggie was "in a daze," as his grandfather, Isaiah, was pointing out. He needed an outlet to deal with the loss of his brother and the pressure he was facing. But as a big, strong black man born into a tough neighborhood in an even tougher world, Reggie, like his brother, wouldn't begin to know how or where to ask for that kind of help.

THE ALL-AMERICA TRAGEDY OF DON ROGERS

Some say the shortest distance between two points can be a spiral. . . .

As if on cue, agents runner Terry Bolar, financier of bachelor parties and limousines, reemerged. Only now, there was no question who he was working for: Agents Norby Walters and Lloyd Bloom of the Walters and Bloom Agency of Manhattan.

Bolar is the agent's liaison who looks and acts like the kids he's trying to recruit. He's black. He played ball. He stands 6-foot-6. He grew up poor. He speaks their language; but most importantly, he seems to understand.

Perhaps soon, people will learn how big a part Bolar played in the Rogers' misery, but at that time, he was just there to help—or maybe he felt guilty. Nevertheless, he could see that Reggie needed something. Bolar is human, he must've sensed that need like a shark smells blood in the water. Swimming circles around Reggie, he assured Reggie that he only wanted what was best for him and that, most importantly, he was there as a friend.

Sure, Terry can fix it. Terry can fix everything.

Then, as they'd done so many times before, either Bolar—or Walters—took out an envelope and spread 5,000 large on the Rogers' living-room floor, covering everything in lifesaving green.

On some level, Reggie probably knew this moment was coming, and maybe he should have severed the relationship long ago. But when you are from The Heights, where nothing is easy, you don't cut benefactors loose without a good reason.

As for Bolar, this moment was the culmination of all the time he'd invested from Day One, and the plan had come together. Some people are born to schmooze. He had found his mark a year before Don died, and part of him surely wanted to bask in his own success. Reggie was a cash cow, and $5,000 was a very cheap price.

Reggie needed a mentor with his best interests at heart—someone like Don. But no one was there. Despite everything that had led him to that very moment, the only immediate concern in Reggie's world was *money*.

Tony Kornheiser of the *Washington Post* called athletic eligibility the "deity" of college sports—sacred, holy, divine. Once it's gone, it's gone forever. And that sin stared Reggie in the face as he looked over all that cash. The conflict surely bore itself before a decision was made; and surely, Bolar was ready to counter any objection.

I'm breaking the rules.
But you're helping your family.
Think of all the headlines if I get caught.
A small sacrifice to bridge this gap.
What if I put Washington on probation?
They make millions off you and don't give you a dime.
I don't know.

Nothing like that's going to happen, Reggie. Everyone's doing this. Let me help you take care of your family. Hell, we'll even postdate the contract until after your bowl game. After everything you've been through, why should you continue to risk everything for free?

Never mind that the following summer the FBI would interrogate Bolar to ascertain whether he gave Don that fatal dose of cocaine. Nor did it matter then that they would later learn who financed Bolar's employers—financiers who enforced their sketchy contracts by any means necessary, whether five dollars or $5,000 was on that living-room floor.

Bolar wasn't lying about one thing, though: Walters and Bloom, aka new agents on the block, were paying college stars left and right. By the time the FBI would uncover everything, cocaine, the day's hot-button topic, and who gave it to Don Rogers would be little less than the tip of the iceberg.

As just yet, however, none of that mattered. All that mattered to Reggie was the money, and whether taking it was the right thing to do. All amateurs hesitate with cash on the table because they all know it's wrong; but without "Uncle" Terry and his envelope of cash, Reggie was up a creek with no paddle.

Besides, in the real world, everyone can use some extra money—especially when that person's sister and mother have no breadwinner.

Don't worry, no one will know. This guy does it. So does this guy. And they're first-rounders.

THE ALL-AMERICA TRAGEDY OF DON ROGERS

The list rolling off Bolar's silver tongue began to seduce Reggie. Sure, The Heights had taught him some street smarts, but nothing about finance—nothing about being the lone chump who says "no" to a chance to help his family.

You could be the first pick in the draft, Reggie. Everyone's saying that.

Perhaps Reggie didn't understand that he was the prize, the object of Bolar's desire. Perhaps the fact that $5,000 was a small price to pay to represent him escaped him as well. But he needed that money. Never mind that a few more months would save his proverbial soul—that, in a few more months, every agent in America would come calling. In December 1986, no laws prohibited agents from wooing players—they only prohibited players from talking to agents. But by the time the good guys would come calling, Reggie's desperation had left them too little, too late.

A rush surely overcame Bolar as his prey scooped up the cash and held it in his hands. Winning at all costs defines those who have failed to achieve their goals fairly. Despite falling short of stardom himself, Bolar now owned a piece of Reggie for life. He'd just made the big time.

Okay, Reggie. Just sign here. We'll make sure this is postdated to cover you.

Reggie now belonged to the Walters and Bloom Agency of Manhattan, or whatever it was being called that week.

No one would ever know.

The 22-year-old man was living in the moment. Taking care of a brokenhearted mother and his downtrodden sister were all that was real to him. He had made the decision to bridge the gap, but the problem was, he had no way to see where that bridge would lead. Such is the way of the desperate youth with an empty room across the hall.

What he couldn't see was, by taking that money he'd notarized his deal with the devil.

18

For days after signing the illegal contract, Reggie couldn't sleep. Wracked with guilt, he contacted a Seattle-based sports attorney named G. Patrick Healy. According to reports, Healy knew Walters and Bloom, and he correctly told Reggie that, by accepting the money, he had made a huge mistake—one that only Healy could fix. Healy told Reggie that everything would be okay, that he'd give Reggie the money to reimburse Walters and Bloom, with interest. He reportedly also told Reggie that nothing was illegal about their transaction.

But that, like most of what Reggie had been eating, was another spoon-fed lie.

When Reggie paid back Bolar's employers, someone—right then and there, whether Walters, Bloom, or Bolar—may have reminded him that he'd signed a contract they wouldn't let him break. No warning, however, could have prepared Reggie for what was to come. At the time, Reggie had no money to sue for—not yet. He didn't understand that these people wouldn't take "no" for an answer. Several star athletes from universities nationwide would soon discover that same thing; but until then, Walters and Bloom were content to bide their time until draft day.

Reggie returned to school for the Sun Bowl, where Washington was thrashed by All-America defensive end Cornelius Bennett and Alabama, 28-6. Though the Huskies finished a respectable 7-5, they were ultimately disappointed after blowing out Ohio State in the season opener.

ONE MOMENT CHANGES EVERYTHING

Blaine Pascal once said, "The whole ocean is affected by a pebble." Had Reggie been able to wait a few more weeks, everything might have turned out differently. *Everything.*

First, a few days after Reggie accepted Healy's loan, Don's insurance settlement arrived. It was no goldmine, but it was more than enough to bridge the Rogers family until April and the NFL draft, in which Reggie was predicted to go between the third and seventh picks overall—a dozen slots higher than Don.

No matter—it was time to celebrate. Despite all that'd happened over the past six months, Reggie's time had come. Even though he was each opponent's top priority on each snap—one game film shows four men attempting to block him on one play—he recorded seven sacks, five forced fumbles, and 100 tackles.

Honors soon followed:

> *First team All-West Coast*
> *First team All-Pac-10 Conference*
> *First team All-America UPI*
> *First team All-America Walter Camp*
> *First team All-America Scripps Howard*
> *First team All-America* The Sporting News
> *First team All-America* The Associated Press
> *First team All-America Football Coaches and Football Writers of America*

Reggie also received the Morris trophy as the Pac-10's most outstanding lineman and was a finalist for the Outland and Lombardi trophies. In addition to being Washington's MVP, his teammates gave him the Guy Flaherty Award, which is given to Washington's most inspirational player.

Rarely is the best player on a team voted the squad's most inspirational teammate. But everyone knew what Reggie had been through, and to see him persevere and then thrive on the field made their decision obvious. Oddly enough, this time, winning an award because of Don was okay for Reggie, as if purity existed behind that single recognition.

THE ALL-AMERICA TRAGEDY OF DON ROGERS

In January 1987, Reggie played in the East-West Shrine All-Star Game in Palo Alto, which included a pregame visit to the Shriners Hospital for Children, where Reggie was a big hit with the kids. He then returned to Seattle for the 52nd annual *Seattle Post-Intelligencer* Star of the Year Award, which is given to the Seattle-area athlete or coach who has had the most impactive year. Coincidentally, Christian Welp, Reggie's replacement and Pac-10 basketball player of the year, is one of the other five finalists.

So, in spite of the tragedy, optimism was smiling down on the Rogers family. Once again, somewhere, perhaps Don was smiling down upon Reggie as well. But if Don was watching, then he could see what was coming. One has to wonder if Reggie felt Don's warnings as he neared the cliff's edge.

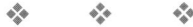

What Reggie needed was a proper agent. Feeling obligated, he briefly signed with Healy, who was president of Professional Sports Management, Inc. Then, thinking Healy was only in it for the money, Reggie reconsidered soon thereafter, firing Healy in lieu of Chicago-based super-agent Steve Zucker, whose clientele included quarterback Jim McMahon and, soon, Deion Sanders.

Normal pre-draft prognostication filled the morning papers as the big day approached, and Tampa Bay, which had the first pick, was sure to take Vinny Testaverde. Rumors arose that the Green Bay Packers, who held the fourth pick, had interest in selecting Reggie to anchor their defense. They'd sent scouts to Seattle to meet with him several times—phoning him nearly every day—and had spoken to his coaches often.

Don James gave Green Bay a glowing recommendation, telling scouts that Reggie was more prepared to play NFL ball than any player he'd ever coached.

"A lot of guys have to do this or that before they're ready, but [Reggie] can have an impact now," attested a coach who, in nine years as Washington's head man, had seen 59 Huskies chosen in NFL drafts.

ONE MOMENT CHANGES EVERYTHING

On April 28, 1987, while Reggie accompanied agent Steve Zucker to the Chicago draft headquarters, reporters gathered at the Rogers' Del Paso Heights home: The house that Don built. Loretha rose at 4:30 a.m. to prepare herself for them, and many will describe her charming makeup and perfectly pressed flower dress. Some correspondents noted the Rose Bowl ring on her index finger and how often she would stop to ponder it.

According to reports, Jackie was nowhere to be found that morning, and no one asked about her. Just five years earlier, Jackie was as well known as her brothers. Although rumors swirled that she'd enrolled in broadcast school, which would have been ideal for such a quick-witted and attractive woman, they were never confirmed.

Facing the television in a large recliner, amidst numerous plaques and trophies and pictures, Loretha—to no one in particular—announced commandingly, "Reggie is going to get his degree."

It was still dark on the West Coast as live coverage began on the draft, and the reporters in attendance were there to *observe* Loretha as much as to conduct interviews. The guests didn't appear to bother her, but she seemed preoccupied, like someone who is alone. Occasionally, she would murmur to herself and sigh, allowing her inner thoughts to be heard by all. The camera's bright light, illuminating her every move, didn't seem to annoy her, either. In fact, as the pre-draft speculation unfolded on TV, she fell asleep more than once.

As though she sensed who was picking, when the Packers were about to choose, Loretha perked up and said, "I know Don would've been wherever Reggie was today. They would've shared this."

Yet, Green Bay passed on Reggie, instead selecting Auburn fullback Brent Fullwood. In reaction, Loretha mumbled, "Don't send Reggie to the snow."

When the No. 7 slot came, NFL commissioner Pete Rozelle announced Reggie as Detroit's first-round pick. Loretha clapped lazily before being interrupted by the phone.

"You like that, Pooh?" she answered. She and Reggie then spoke about their love for each other, about how everything would now be okay.

Hanging up, she turned to the reporters. "Any time Reggie is happy, I'm happy," she told them.

"I know Don is there in Chicago with Reggie right now," she said, clearing her throat. "I just know it."

As the seventh overall pick, Reggie became the highest selection ever from the University of Washington. Detroit was smart to choose him, he told reporters, because they'd be getting two players in one: Don and himself.

Eyebrows had risen because the Packers, desperate for defensive linemen, had passed on Reggie, who many considered the best available player in his entry class. A few weeks later, a report surfaced, claiming that the Packers had hired a private investigator to tail Reggie. Supposedly, they found some of the information troubling. "You wouldn't believe what we found out about the guy," Packers personnel director Tom Braatz allegedly told the *Green Bay Press Gazette*. "It was enough to know we shouldn't draft him."

Braatz would later deny making the statement.

Detroit head coach Darryl Rogers asserted that any stories about teams hiring private investigators was utterly false, assuring them that he has never heard of any team going outside the organization to research a player. Though, with millions invested into these young men, not doing so seems foolish; franchises employed dozens of capable people to research draft picks and sift through garbage.

In terms of talent, the 1987 draft is considered reasonably fruitful. Reggie was the third defensive player chosen, behind Alabama's Cornelius Bennett (Indianapolis) and Duke's Mike Junkin (Cleveland). Purdue safety and All-America hurdler Rod Woodson (Pittsburgh) and Heisman runner-up Paul Palmer of Temple (Kansas City) were taken at No. 10 and No. 19, respectively.

All of these young men would be linked together very soon.

ONE MOMENT CHANGES EVERYTHING

Reggie, who was flown to Detroit immediately for press conferences and a Lions mini-camp, sat calmly as GM Russ Thomas introduced him as "Reggie Rucker," who, coincidentally, had played wide receiver for the Cleveland Browns. Without missing a beat, the reporters picked up right where they left off in Seattle. The very first question asked of Reggie and ever-present Steve Zucker involved Don and drugs.

Thomas immediately issued a strong denial and cited the negative results of his pick's drugs tests in his defense. He then clarified his position to mesh with the country's stance, stating, "The unfortunate side of the association will cause people to become more aware of potential problems with Reggie. It's something he is going to have to live with for the rest of his life."

A year after his brother's death, and still Reggie was paying for something Don had done to himself. When pushed to respond the day after the draft, Reggie said, "Today's a pretty happy day in my life, and I don't want to get into that."

Pausing, he then said, "I just know Don's happy."

After mini-camp, the entire Lions staff was beaming over Reggie's potential. "Reggie is an excellent athlete, and he proved that at camp," said head coach Darryl Rogers. "He's big and strong and a great football player. By far, [he is] the best pass rusher in the draft."

The drug questions weren't going away, though. In May, a reporter questioned how Reggie planned to keep himself drug-free. He replied:

> "This thing is like a black cloud hanging over my head. It's not my fault. I didn't do it. That gets [put] next to me when people ask me how I'm going to prevent drugs from happening to me. It's unfair. I'm here, and I've promised so many people I'm never going to do this. I'm never going to do that. Hey, I'm 23 years old; and it's like my whole life is based on 'nots.' Sometimes, there seems so little space to grow."

THE ALL-AMERICA TRAGEDY OF DON ROGERS

Meanwhile, as Congress began work on even tougher drug laws, the NCAA uncovered a scandal involving Rod Woodson, Cris Carter, Reggie Rogers, and several others that would rival the drug war altogether.

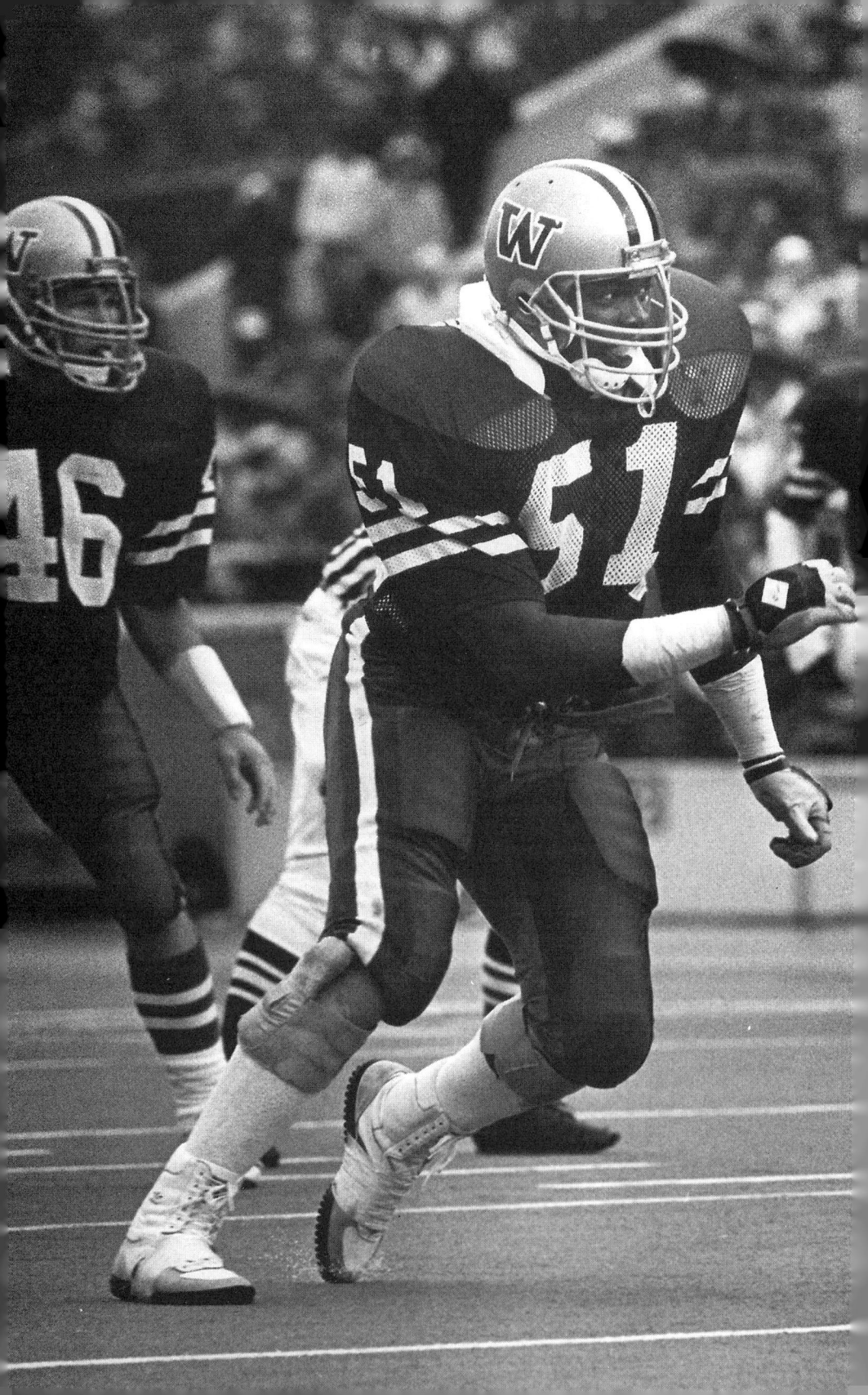

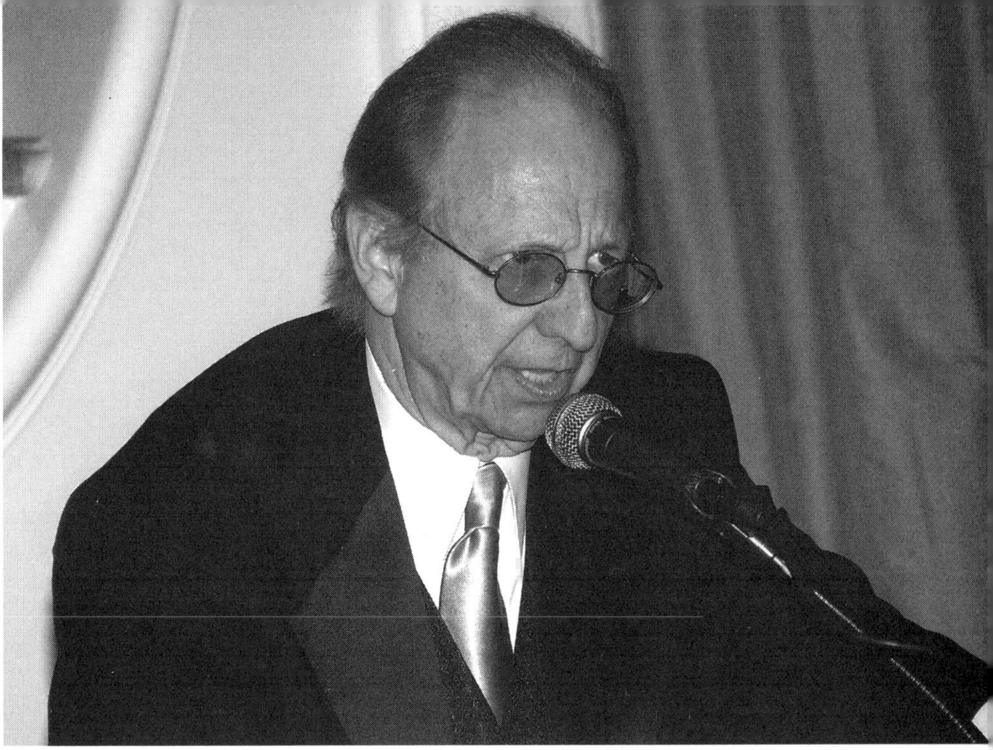

Left: Reggie Rogers (51) in action as a Washington Husky.
Photo courtesy of the University of Washington Athletic Department
Above: Super agent Norby Walters in 2006. *Photo by Stephen Shugerman/Getty Images*
Below: Jackie Rogers visits the graves of her mother, Loretha, and brother, Don, on the 20th anniversary of Don's death. *Photo courtesy of* The Sacramento Bee

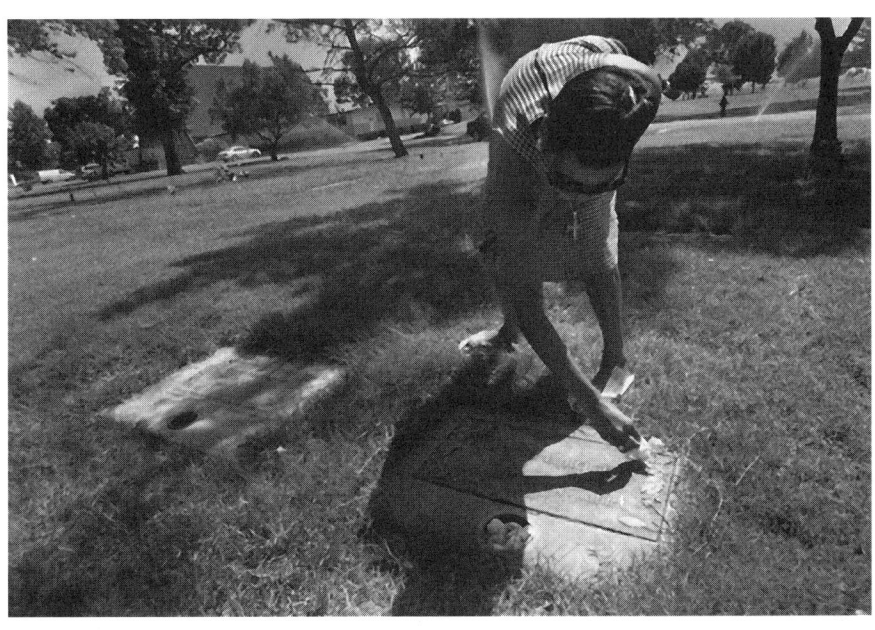

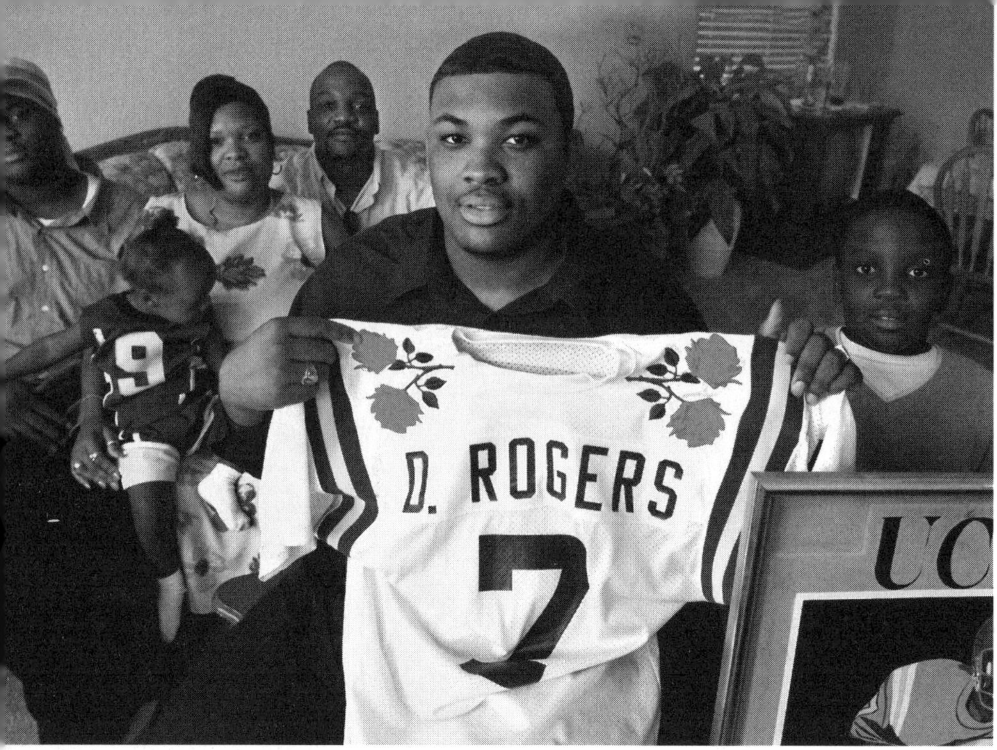

Above: Also known as "Little D," Don Rogers Jr.—surrounded by his family—proudly displays his father's Rose Bowl jersey. *Photo courtesy of* The Sacramento Bee

Below: Don Rogers' grave marker. *Photo courtesy of* The Sacramento Bee

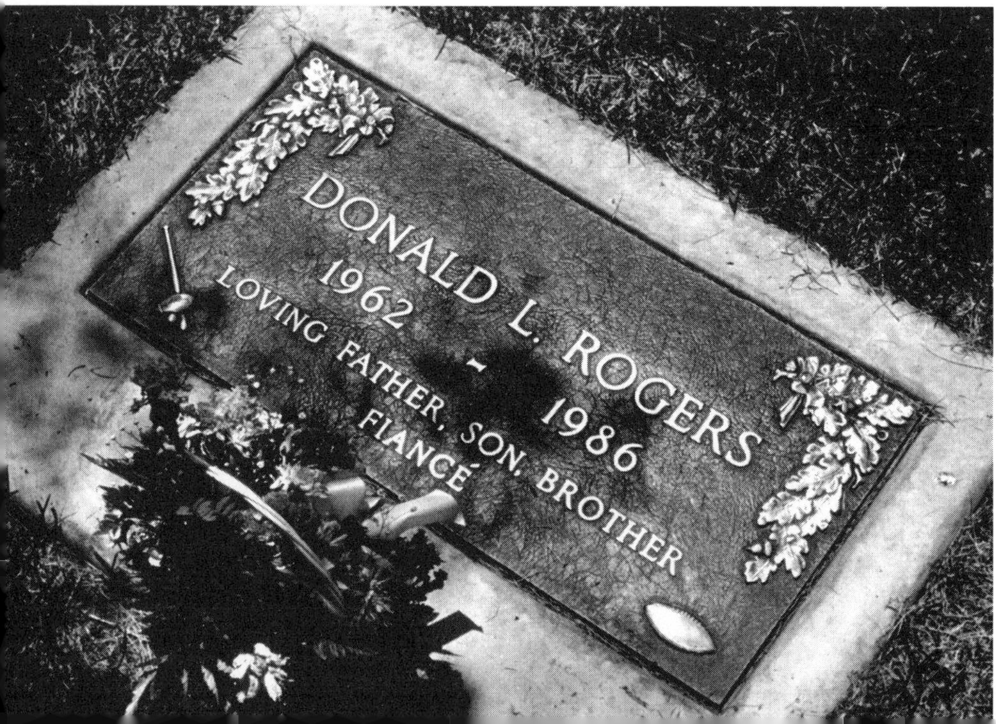

19

The biggest stories often start small. Though the war on drugs may have begun in the early '80s, the movement didn't hit stride until Len Bias and Don died in 1986. Not as notorious or far-reaching as the drug war, a story appeared in *The New York Times* and the *Chicago Tribune* that reported an anonymous football player had lodged a complaint against the Walters and Bloom Agency—specifically, Norby Walters—for "threatening to break his legs" after he had fired Walters. Overlooked initially, that article would rock the NCAA and all of college sports at its very foundation.

Before founding a sports agency, Norby Walters was in the entertainment business, owning several nightclubs in New York City. As an entertainment executive, Walters had his share of success, even managing such performers as Dionne Warwick and Marvin Gaye. Some believed that he had much help in securing management positions, though, and that the mafia determined when and how far Walters could climb the entrepreneurial ladder.

According to some early 1980s testimony, Walters reportedly convinced notorious Colombo crime family captain Michael Franzese to invest in his newest endeavor: World Sports and Entertainment. Walters had known Franzese's father, another Colombo captain, for 40 years, but by the age of 23, Michael had become one of the biggest names in mafia history.

Vanity Fair called him "The prince of the mafia."

"The biggest earner since Al Capone," said *Fortune Magazine*.

One of the Colombo Crime Family's primary sources of revenue was gambling. Franzese was rumored to bring in as much as $1 million per week through illegal gambling alone. So when Walters proposed a sports agency, Franzese and his associates realized that would give them the ability to "coerce" athletes into altering games by shaving points to the Mafioso's satisfaction. For decades, the mafia had known that the best way to gain control of athletes was to pay them while they were still in college, setting them up for blackmail when the time was right.

In March 1987, a *Chicago Tribune* article said the National Football League Players Association was investigating Walters' dealings with several players preparing for the April 28 draft. Two unnamed players had been represented by Walters briefly but were now under contract to agent Steve Zucker. Each had told the NFLPA that someone had called threatening to "break my legs" for firing Walters.

A week later, *The New York Times* reported startling new developments: The FBI was now investigating an early-morning March 16 assault that had taken place at Steve Zucker's headquarters. Kathe Clements, a vice president at Zucker Sports Entertainment Group and wife of Canadian Football League star Tom Clements, had arrived early for work. A masked man appeared from nowhere and beat her unconscious before slashing her arm with a knife. The attack followed weeks of ominous phone calls placed to Zucker's office, as well as to the two former Walters clients—now identified as Nebraska running back Doug Dubose and Washington defensive end Reggie Rogers.

"If the guy wanted to kill her, he probably could have," said Skokie police lieutenant Michael Langer. "Somebody sent them a message, there is no doubt about that."

For his part, Walters never even attempted to conceal the fact that he'd paid college athletes. No laws prohibited his end of the deal, which apparently made it open season. When questioned about the players' accusations, he issued the following denial: "Sickening, really sickening—who knows what these kids will say to break their contracts?"

The day after the NFL draft, Norby's name was back in the *New York Times*. He was claiming to have signed representation agreements with seven of the 28 first-round picks—breaking super-agent Leigh Steinberg's record of four, set the previous year.

"Isn't that amazing," Walters told the *Times*. "For a guy to get seven first-rounders is really humongous. I'm some picker, aren't I?"

Though most of those players saw things differently, Walters was unfettered. He instructed his attorney, Lonn Trost, to file lawsuits alleging breach of contract against five of those seven picks, including Rod Woodson, Brent Fullwood, Terrence Flagler, Tony Woods, and Reggie Rogers. The remaining two clients, John Clay and Paul Palmer, had decided to continue their professional relationship with Walters and Bloom. For reasons unknown, only Walters' lawsuits against Fullwood, Woods, Flagler, and Woodson included signed promissory notes for loans dating back before their senior seasons. Whether because he only had one game left to play or because he paid back the loan with interest, the lawsuit against Reggie contained no such documentation, only the assertion that he'd breached his contract.

When prodded to comment on the Clements beating investigation, Walters claimed that several agents were conspiring to drive him out of the business due to his success, telling reporters, "This will all go away." Two days later, Dallas' FBI office announced that it had voice recordings of Walters' partner, Lloyd Bloom, threatening SMU wide receiver Ronald Morris. Supposedly, Bloom told Morris someone would break his hand if he signed with any other agent—but no mention of the purported recordings ever surfaced again.

Meanwhile, Reggie's agent problems were actually intensifying. G. Patrick Healy, who'd loaned him money to pay back Walters and Bloom, jumped on the lawsuit bandwagon and sued Reggie and Steve Zucker for breach of contract. In return, Reggie retained attorneys, who sued both Walters and Healy for a combined $2.7 million in damages for using fraud and duress to secure his contract.

Matters were complicated further in early June—almost a full year after Don's death—when the FBI revealed they were investigating whether Walters and Bloom employee Terry Bolar had supplied the cocaine that killed Don Rogers. Responding to the allegations, Bolar supposedly replied, "I didn't have anything to do with any drugs and Don. I'll put my hand on many stacks of Bibles and swear on it."

A grand jury was convened in Chicago to inspect Walters and Bloom. Although the government was anxious to create a case against World Sports and Entertainment—and their financial backers, the Colombo crime family—they had no evidence in the Clements beating other than the possible threats. Nor did prosecutors have concrete evidence on Don's cocaine-induced death. And, since paying amateur athletes was not yet illegal, the FBI was limited in what charges they could pursue. Yet, just as Al Capone was nailed for tax evasion instead of rackets and murder, a creative federal prosecutor built the argument that, by paying amateur athletes, Walters and Bloom had committed fraud against the corresponding universities.

The problem was, if the FBI pursued the agency, they also might have to pursue the athletes, who committed their own fraud by misrepresenting their incomes to receive scholarship financial aid. No one was going to admit to tens of thousands in under-the-table payoffs or weekly cash stipends. Authorities didn't want to prosecute the athletes, though; they simply needed their testimony. Still, all the athletes had reservations.

One way around prosecution was to grant the athletes immunity as State's witnesses; but coercion was no less involved there, and testifying still placed them in grave danger.

In all, 40 football players from 20 different universities and their corresponding scholarship documentation were subpoenaed.

Meanwhile, the issue had created backlash in other areas. Ohio State All-America wide receiver Cris Carter, just a junior, was ruled ineligible when NCAA officials learned that he'd accepted a $5,000 advance and monthly payments from Walters and Bloom. Rod Woodson's track career at Purdue, as well as his Olympic dreams, disintegrated when the case was made public. Derrick

THE ALL-AMERICA TRAGEDY OF DON ROGERS

McKey, an All-America junior basketball player at Alabama, lost his eligibility for similar transgressions involving the W&B Agency.

Yet Reggie had his own problems. Caught in a legal crossfire and in debt to the mafia, he had just learned that the man he brought into his mother's home—into his brother's home—may have played a role in his brother's death. The taxing pressure was mounting each day.

To deal, Reggie began consuming large quantities of alcohol.

20

One year after her son had died, Lonise Bias was well on her way to becoming a highly sought drug consultant and motivational speaker. People lined up to hear her story anywhere she went. She was awarded an honorary doctorate of education from Anna Maria College in Massachusetts. Turning her tragedy into a victory of sorts, thousands will attest to Lonise's positive influence on their lives. Yet that outpour would not insulate her from further heartbreak—she would lose another son, Jay, in a 1990 drive-by shooting. Deluged by interview requests, Loretha had to change her phone number several times to fend off reporters looking for a fresh way to view her son's death on its one-year anniversary.

Washington Post columnist Michael Wilbon commemorated "the day a lot of people grew up" in East Coast fashion, writing not remembrances of Bias or Don, but a sober recap of cocaine's toll on athletics over the previous year.

"If Don Rogers could die just eight days after Bias," Wilbon pondered, "how much wiser are we?"

Wilbon also noted that World Champion New York Mets star pitcher Dwight Gooden, who, in 1984, had become the youngest All-Star ever at 19, had just entered rehab. He also pointed out that the NBA had suspended Walter Davis, Lewis Lloyd, and Mitchell Wiggins, perhaps forever, for cocaine use. From the 1986 NBA draft alone—which included Bias—Roy Tarpley, Chris Washburn, and William Bedford would have their careers derailed by cocaine as well. Nearer to Wilbon's D.C. office, he observed that the once proud University of Maryland was freefalling. Not only had basketball coach Lefty Driesell been forced out—he had told an assistant coach, Oliver Purnell, to "clean up Bias' room," and Purnell refused—but the Terrapins football coach had resigned due to the school's tarnished reputation.

Across the country, newspapers on the West Coast—*The Los Angeles Times, San Francisco Chronicle, Sacramento Union* and *Sacramento Bee* all commemorated the anniversary with the same questions and concerns, only with Don in the lead. The *Union* ran an article in which a reporter asked whether the excruciating pain that locals felt over losing Don would ever subside. Interviews with residents around Del Paso Heights revealed grief-stricken fans and friends of Don who apparently were nowhere close to accepting that the first son of The Heights was gone forever.

"He was idolized by just about everyone in Del Paso Heights," said Grant High School Principal Bill Crenshaw in a *Sacramento Bee* interview. "Donald would always say, 'You've got to stay in school.' He'd say, 'Education is a way of out of Del Paso Heights; you can go anywhere you want.' He had money, but he never flaunted it—you just knew it by the way he carried himself."

The *Bee* ran a multipage account of the previous year: the aftermath of Don's death, the introduction of drug testing, new drug sentencing laws, and rising incarceration rates. Also included were Reggie's highlights and lowlights: his quick ascension to football's elite, his All-America recognitions, becoming the seventh pick in the NFL draft, lawsuits, payoff accusations, and mob-connected former agents.

Some lack the capacity to put Don's death in perspective, though. In another article, a paragraph details Little D's recent birthday party—his first without his father. Evidently, he spent most of the evening waiting for Don to walk through the front door carrying presents. "He doesn't know," Loretha told a reporter solemnly as they gazed down upon Little D nibbling pizza. After a "period of isolation," Loretha had taken an active role in managing the Pop Warner football team Don and Reggie had founded, the North Sacramento Browns.

THE ALL-AMERICA TRAGEDY OF DON ROGERS

In examining who had supplied the cocaine that killed Don, the *Bee* noted the Sacramento Police Department had suspected "a local person" of the crime, contradicting previously published reports that Terry Bolar was the primary suspect. A Sacramento Police Department spokesperson said, "The self-induced nature of the death and the absence of witnesses make prosecution impractical." Perhaps the FBI had implicated Bolar merely to shake down his employers.

Ironically, each article chronicled minute-by-minute timelines of the morning of Don's death, how Loretha and Little D had been dealing as well as Reggie's rollercoaster year; but none of them made any mention of Jackie, as though she'd vanished altogether.

The anniversary was more for the papers than the Rogers, though. Each time a law was changed, a milestone was reached, an athlete entered rehab, or someone connected to Don was interviewed, the Rogers family phone would start ringing. In Detroit, Reggie's new home; the media would mention Don nearly as much as the city's newest star, as if Reggie were the surviving Siamese twin following sacrificial surgery.

Despite his undisputed talent, Reggie was having trouble treading rough waters away from the field, and fans in Detroit seemed to expect him to drown.

The Lions, however, decided enough was enough. Too much negative media attention was focused on Reggie, who'd begun to show obvious signs of strain, snapping at reporters during interviews. Unlike the University of Washington's handlers, the Lions circled their wagons around their rookie defensive end. Thus, Reggie could only give interviews in the Lion offices, and only if a team official was present.

The Lions' coaches, however, were ecstatic about Reggie's potential. "Even if we'd had the first pick in the draft, we'd have chosen Reggie," said one team spokesperson. "We got the player we wanted most."

Despite the team's vigilance, however, unfiltered Reggie quotes soon found their way into the Detroit papers anyway. Anyone who'd followed the past year of his life could tell that he was beginning to feel victimized. When one reporter asked about his fracas with agents, he replied, "Is this 'Pick on Reggie' year or something?"

Those paying attention had to admit that Reggie had been through hell, but his pity party wasn't what people looking for heroes and role models wanted to hear. Referring to himself in the third person wasn't helping, either.

"This didn't start until my brother died," he would later say, responding to his run of bad luck. "Everything started to go downhill as soon as he died. Every day, something happened."

After just one regular-season game—one in which Reggie recorded a sack but also made a blitzing mistake that led to a long Minnesota Vikings touchdown—an article appeared in the *Sacramento Bee* that took Reggie's budding persecution complex a step further. The writer quoted Reggie as saying he felt "abused" by his coaches, who didn't understand him. He believed that they should just cut him loose and let him play, as he was allowed to do in college.

Though the reporter went on to write that Detroit's coaches had every confidence in Reggie, who they were sure would be an NFL star; a glaring journalistic error haunted the article. A color photograph of Reggie, handsome and smiling, accompanied the piece. Beneath the picture was a caption that read: "Don Rogers of the Detroit Lions."

Walls were closing in on Reggie: lawsuits, anonymous phone calls warning him not to testify against Walters and Bloom, Loretha's worsening heart trouble. Battling minor injuries, Reggie was splitting time at defensive end when, to everyone's dismay, the NFL Players Association voted to go on strike. While NFL owners scrambled to field teams of replacement players so they could satisfy their television contracts, the downtime was bad for everyone, especially Reggie. This 23-year-old man, who had experienced more stress in his young life than most families do in consecutive generations, was left to fend for himself in a strange city.

Then Jackie got back into the mix. She flew to Detroit to visit her brother. One day, she borrowed Reggie's truck—but didn't come back. Hours passed, then a full day with no word. Two days elapsed, and Reggie was frantic. After he filed a missing-person report, he got a call from police: There was a body in the morgue that could be Jackie.

The body turned out to be another unfortunate missing girl; so Reggie, at once relieved and panicked, took to driving the city's streets, desperately looking for his sister. *The New York Times*, the *Detroit Free Press*, the Sacramento papers, Chicago, every rag ran a story on the missing Rogers girl, and volunteers began canvassing Detroit.

After being gone for four full days without word, Jackie returned to Reggie's apartment. She insisted that she was with a friend. What could he do but put her on a plane back to Sacramento? In the layover at Chicago's O'Hare Airport, Jackie didn't re-board for the flights second leg, though, and again disappeared. Perhaps Reggie knew all along; but reportedly, a family member finally informed Reggie that Jackie was addicted to cocaine.

It was all just too much. . . . Reggie finally hit the wall.

A headline in the *Chicago Tribune* would read, "Rogers In Toughest Battle Yet."

Reports appeared in newspapers across the land that said: "The Detroit Lions have placed Reggie Rogers on the non-football related injured reserve list."

Loretha soon had to inform the media that Reggie was suffering a nervous breakdown. He entered a Pontiac-area emotional counseling center; but once again, the press went to great lengths to connect Reggie, who had two siblings associated with drugs, to cocaine.

Neither the Lions nor Reggie's spokesperson could issue denials quick enough to match the onslaught of accusations. Though Reggie had passed every drug test—and the hard truth was, he was not on drugs—he readily admitted that he sought care for alcohol dependency during his counseling.

When the strike ended, Reggie returned to the Lions after a 30-day stay in the treatment facility and played the final two regular-season games. The Detroit media, though, was on "Reggie Watch." Many people were claiming that Reggie was a complete bust, and the Detroit coaching staff wasn't refuting those opinions as often as they could have.

Everyone agreed that the off-season was going to be very long and very important for Reggie Rogers.

21

By early May 1988, the noose was tightening around sports agents Norby Walters and Lloyd Bloom. Atop the FBI investigations, individual states had begun to prosecute them as well. Alabama was the first to gain a settlement, as they trapped Bloom into admitting to a misdemeanor charge of deceptive trade practices. Yet, in return for dropping commercial bribery charges, Alabama authorities had convinced Bloom to testify against Walters.

Cases of that nature—extortion, threats, bribery, blackmail—depend on extensive witness corroboration and testimony and, without a paper trail or a corpse, are quite difficult to prosecute. Expert defense attorneys can rattle witnesses, turning testimony upside down.

The trials against the agents were far from slam dunks.

In June, the state of Alabama agreed to drop charges against Walters in exchange for a $200,000 fine and a signed promise that Walters would never interfere with eligible student-athletes attending any Southeastern Conference school. Money aside, it was a slap on the wrist; but the settlement was a sign of things to come.

The Walters and Bloom pay-and-blackmail scandals reverberated around the country. Because running back Paul Palmer admitted to accepting Walters' money while still at Temple, the university agreed to forfeit all six wins from the 1986 season. Then all Palmer's records were expunged, all his awards were overturned, and he still had to repay his advances.

ONE MOMENT CHANGES EVERYTHING

The player suffered, and the university was embarrassed, but how did that punish the targets of the probe?

The FBI failed to compile any evidence linking Terry Bolar to the cocaine that killed Don. Unlike the Len Bias case—where his best friend, Brian Tribble, was put on trial for supplying the cocaine—no further evidence would appear.

No arrests were made in the death of Don Rogers. No arrests will ever be made.

In the end, 43 athletes who concealed or lied about receiving payments were assigned community service, required to pay back any scholarship money they defrauded from their universities (28 in all), and most importantly, had to testify against Walters and Bloom. The U.S. government ultimately wanted to reveal the agency's link to the Colombo Crime Family, but in their overzealousness, prosecutors had created a case with no existing precedent on little hard evidence. Despite that fact, federal authorities formally charged Walters and Bloom with racketeering, conspiracy, mail fraud, wire fraud, and a single count of extortion—but they found zero proof that Kathe Clements was attacked at their behest.

If convicted, Walters and Bloom faced up 70 years in prison and millions in fines. But as the investigation progressed, the FBI uncovered several compelling rumors, but too few could be confirmed. The government alleged that, as far back as 1981, Walters and Michael Franzese—who, by now, has become a born-again Christian—had approached the (Michael) Jackson Five threatening to cancel their world tour if Walters wasn't hired as the group's booking agent. But again, no real proof existed, and people who had gotten on with their lives, who prospered, had little to gain by testifying against known mafia associates.

The grand jury indicted only one athlete, former Ohio State wide receiver Cris Carter, who, by then—via a special supplemental draft that Carter would've missed had he retained eligibility—was a member of the Philadelphia Eagles. Carter was accused of obstruction of justice for denying he received payments, and of mail fraud for using U.S. postal offices to send illegal contracts. His reluctance to admit his involvement made some sense, for, at the time of his initial interrogation, he was one of the few players in question who had eligibility remaining. Threatened with 10 years in prison and a $500,000 fine, Carter pled guilty. On the condition he would cooperate with federal prosecutors, he agreed to community service.

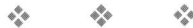

As Reggie prepared for his highly anticipated sophomore effort in Detroit, positive news emerged. He was abstaining from alcohol, embracing religion, and finding love—Reggie had become engaged to one Sheila Dorsey. He seemed to have become a forthright, contemplative young man who was facing his demons. His defensive attitude had been replaced with earnestness and humility. The press wanted as much face time with him as possible, and Reggie wasn't backing down from tough questions.

Everyone agreed that a lack of talent or intellect was not Reggie's problem. The young man was engaging and, at times, had reporters and teammates cracking up with his sharp sense of humor. On the field, coaches shook their heads, marveling at his combination of size—after an off-season spent in the weight room, he now weighed 290—strength, and finesse.

In what must have seemed like a twisted cosmic joke, the Lions' first two preseason games of the 1988 slate were at Cleveland and at home against the Seattle Seahawks. That meant the reporters who covered those teams were intimately familiar with Reggie and his family history. Following the Seattle game, Reggie was asked to respond to a pre-training camp quote attributed to Detroit coach Darryl Rogers, who'd reportedly told him, "Improve or you're gone."

Reggie calmly deliberated for several moments, then replied, "I've had a lot of problems. To be honest with you, the problems are still here right now; and they will probably still be with me when I'm done playing football."

ONE MOMENT CHANGES EVERYTHING

Perhaps those reporters who couldn't determine "why" Reggie had done so many things wrong were settling back on their heels a bit just then. Maybe they allowed their shoulders to slump and put their accusations to rest. Maybe they even felt a little shame.

Maybe.

Reggie is only human. His hero and guiding light had perished; and depression, accompanied by acute substance sensitivity, ran through his genes the way brown hair or green eyes did for other people.

"I've got my priorities straight now," he added.

Although those same men were paid to prod Reggie about drug and alcohol abuse, about his agent problems, one has to wonder whether they were pulling for him, just a bit. Surely, they hoped that he would get his act together so his story would have a happy ending. The better Reggie played, the more they could enjoy their jobs.

After that Seahawks preseason game, Lions head coach Darryl Rogers told the same media, "Reggie's played the best he ever played for us. This year, he's done everything he's supposed to. He's a much better player. He's what we thought he was when we drafted him."

Nothing beats a redemption story, after all—especially when witnessing one that ends in greatness.

A July 18 article in *The Sporting News* had quoted Reggie admitting he had become a heavy drinker since Don's death, and he addressed his stay at a Detroit counseling center.

"How can I have so much and still be so depressed?," he recalled asking the staff.

Then, when discussing his first NFL season, his poor start, the strike, and the ensuing downtime, he said, "The only thing keeping me together was football, and then my football was getting all messed up."

If the story of the Rogers family could've ended there, even if Reggie's NFL career was merely average, that would've been more than enough. Several talented, unsophisticated young men encounter legal trouble with unscrupulous sports agents. Many

THE ALL-AMERICA TRAGEDY OF DON ROGERS

families face drug abuse. In 1988, though, the saga of Sacramento's First Family of Athletes was still unfolding.

And in October, it would take a horrific, deadly turn.

After the season's first month, Reggie wasn't tearing up the league, but he was showing signs of life, making him an early candidate for the Most Improved Player Award. He was working hard, and working harder to shed the burdens of his past.

On October 2, Reggie hurt his ankle against the 49ers, which would sideline him for several weeks. Several callers began to lambaste Detroit talk radio, insisting that Reggie was the biggest bust in NFL history.

But Reggie knew he just needed to heal and get back onto the field. He knew he could be a star and make his brother proud. And he probably felt that, once he reached that level, everything would be okay. *Everything.*

Downtime, however, had never been good for Reggie. Three weeks passed, and his ankle still hadn't healed. His fiancée, Sheila, who was pregnant, was back in Seattle. Battling the desire to drink away his free time, and doing his best to ignore the incessant questions from people wondering whether his ankle would ever mend, Reggie headed out for a drive.

Wherever he intended to go, he ended up at the one place he knew to avoid: Big Art's Paradise Lounge.

The next thing Reggie Rogers knew, he was waking up in a hospital with a broken neck and a severed thumb, his head immobilized in a metal halo. The police soon arrived to inform him that he'd be arrested upon his release from intensive care. Bewildered, he asked a question that had been posed to him for far too long.

"Why? What did I do?"

22

For weeks, drivers would slow down at the intersection of University and Wide Track Drive, hoping to catch a glimpse of the chalk marks and broken glass. Several people laid flowers on the sidewalk nearby. Disaster tourists would arrive from miles around to take "it" all in, gawking at the sterile, bleached-concrete crossroads where lanes are straight and wide, the corners are sharp, and the curbs are severe.

The light was green. No one lives in that area. People sped past at all hours.

At Big Art's, Reggie drank enough to get drunk, then met a young woman who needed a ride home. Teammate Devon Mitchell and his companion were leaving, too, so Reggie and his new friend followed behind them in his Jeep.

Earlier that same morning, somewhere not too far away, Kenneth Willett, 19, and his two cousins—Kelly and Dale Ess, 18 and 17, respectively, who were in town to visit their terminally ill grandmother—apparently woke up with loaded guns to their temples. After visiting their grandma, the three teens went somewhere and they got good and drunk. Most people wouldn't remember that, though; nor would they recall the bag of pot the boys had stashed in their black van.

At approximately 1:50 a.m. that night, there was a collision, then an explosion, then a fireball. The three teens were incinerated and unrecognizable, though not all three died instantly.

Reggie broke his neck in three places, and almost completely severed his thumb. Over the next month, he wouldn't be able to lift his legs, and a tube would be used to clear his throat. His face was slashed, and his front teeth were gone. His passenger survived, but she severed a finger as well.

Right there, right then, and probably rightly so, Reggie's past didn't matter anymore. The forewarning hordes, the accusers, those who bet against him—they were right about him now even though they were wrong.

Again with the front-page news.

Again with the incriminations and social commentary.

Again, Reggie had become an epicenter.

This time it was easy. People got to say, "I told you so," because the big, black, intimidating villain—from a drug-riddled family, no less—stood right in front of them. He'd been in more trouble than anyone had the right to walk away from, but he was rich. Reggie Rogers was no longer just Don Rogers' brother. He'd surpassed Don athletically at comparable stages in their careers. Now, he'd blown past Don in terms of notoriety as well.

Loretha and Joe, though divorced for years, flew cross-country along with Jackie to be with Reggie at Pontiac Osteopathic Hospital. Everyone prayed. While Joe wouldn't speak to the press, Loretha blamed herself. "I was pregnant with his sister right after Reggie was born, and I always felt I wasn't able to give him the attention of a newborn baby," she said.

But no one else would think of that giant in a halo as a baby anymore—not when he had blood on his hands. Lying in a hospital bed, heavily medicated, Reggie drifted in and out of consciousness. "Momma," someone heard him say, "why don't they let Don rest in peace?"

Loretha, as if speaking to her child after a nightmare, replied, "Don't worry, son. Don't worry. Don is with us."

"I'm the one who's got to hold everyone up," Reggie mumbled. "I can't take being like this. I can't take them doing what they're doing to Don."

"After Don's death, Reggie tried to be a father, an uncle, and a brother, never taking care of Reggie," Loretha would later tell *The New York Times*. "He's never made time to deal with Don's death."

THE ALL-AMERICA TRAGEDY OF DON ROGERS

Accounts of the accident varied, but some witnesses would say that the van carrying the three teenagers was at fault. Others would testify that Reggie was to blame. However, only one thing was certain to those who had followed Reggie's career: If he, Jackie, and Loretha hadn't recovered from Don's death, they'd never recover now.

Before his arraignment, Oakland County Prosecutors announced that they would seek three counts of involuntary manslaughter against Reggie—the most severe charges allowed under Michigan law—with each count bringing 15 years in prison. While ample community outrage swelled against Reggie, reports surfaced that the three teenagers were intoxicated and under the legal drinking age. In response, prosecutor L. Brooks Patterson began to build his case in the media, saying: "We will not allow the teenagers to be put on trial."

Soon thereafter, Patterson assured Detroit, "There will be no plea bargaining in this case."

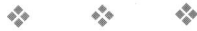

The Rogers family didn't give up however.

"Every day I tell him he's lucky to be alive," Loretha would say, "and to pray for the families that lost their children."

Reggie married his fiancée, Sheila Dorsey, from his hospital bed, then hired celebrity Detroit attorney Elbert Hatchett, who had successfully defended former Detroit Lions star running back Billy Sims in a breach-of-contract lawsuit filed by the Houston Gamblers of the United States Football League. Hatchett was listed as a "Who's Who of Black Millionaires," but was battling the federal government, which demanded he pay more than $3 million in back taxes. Starting his own media blitz, Hatchett told friends and relatives of Reggie, "Keep the faith. Proof will show that he was not culpable."

Lions players were instructed not to talk about the accident, but some did anyway. Popular wide receiver Jeff Chadwick told *The*

ONE MOMENT CHANGES EVERYTHING

New York Times, "We're trying not to let it affect us, but how can we not let it affect us? We think about it, we talk about it."

Journalists nationwide would sit down to pen the epic "Rise and Fall" articles that win awards and prompt readers to reflect over their morning cups of coffee. Back home, in Del Paso Heights, reporters searched for that perfect summation, descending upon North Sacramento only to find that the neighborhood was turning against Reggie. A Grant High School teacher, who viewed the story in stark racial and economic terms, told the *Sacramento Bee*, "You've heard about the extinction of the black male—we need to get as much out of the few of us who are successful. Here's Reggie, who watches the mistakes his brother made, and he falls into the same trap."

Over at Robertson Community Center, though—the Rogers' second home—people weren't ready to abandon Reggie just yet. The day after the accident, kids from the center brought Loretha and Jackie cookies and then mowed their lawn. Just days earlier, Reggie had visited town and taken several North Sacramento Browns to dinner.

"I met Reggie three days before the accident," said a sparkling-eyed player named Edwin in a *Sacramento Bee* interview. "He bought pizzas for everybody. I talked to him and shook his hand. He was a nice guy. He smiled all the time."

With seventh graders, pizza and stardom carried disproportionate weight, as most kids only know they want some of both. In response to the accident's details, though, the child went numb.

"When I showed him the paper with Reggie's smashed Jeep, he read it over and over and over. He couldn't say anything," said Edwin's father, who had worked with Del Paso Heights youth for over 30 years, and worked at Robertson with both Don and Reggie.

When Reggie left the hospital, he was booked into jail immediately. After paying a $10,000 bond, he pled innocent to three counts of involuntary manslaughter, determined to avoid 45 years in prison, on November 14.

THE ALL-AMERICA TRAGEDY OF DON ROGERS

On November 16, Reggie's wife, Sheila, gave birth to twins, Regina and Reggie Jr., thus beginning the next generation of Rogers. Those aware of Don, Reggie, and Jackie—each a modern manifestation of Achilles—surely wondered who the children would ultimately become.

On November 19, Reggie was served with a multimillion-dollar civil suit initiated by the Willett and Ess families.

Forever there for her son, Loretha, although faltering in heart but never in spirit, would tell him, "We're the best team, the best team in the world. One day at a time, Reggie—don't even think football. Just wake up every day and thank God you're alive and not dead."

Though Reggie's attorney had instructed him to remain mum, Jackie spoke openly and provided the defining line all those journalists desperately needed.

"Maybe there's a curse on this family."

23

By spring 1989, the Chicago racketeering trial of Walters and Bloom was in full swing. Chilling testimony from Chicago Bears free safety Maurice Douglass seemed to put one nail in the agents' coffins. After telling them that he wished to sever their business agreement back in 1986, Bloom allegedly told Douglass, "Somebody might break your legs." Like all the other witnesses, though, Douglass was far from snow pure. He admitted to taking up to $10,000 of Walters and Bloom Agency's money while he was still at Kentucky. Awaiting the 1986 NFL Draft at his mother's Cincinnati home, Douglass told the grand jury, Bloom called him several times saying that Douglass wouldn't make it to draft day if he didn't return all the money.

Defense attorneys aptly noted that Bloom's purported threat never materialized, and that Douglass failed to call the police, tell his new agents, or inform his coaches at the University of Kentucky. Then they pointed out that Douglass *did* pay back the loan to Walters and Bloom.

With so many star athletes and insiders lined up as State's witnesses, Reggie Rogers, now lacking credibility, was not called to testify.

If the government were going to win, it would have to do so by proving the agents inflicted damage on either the athletes or the universities. Ultimately, prosecutors were digging for a conviction and a severe sentence that could be used as leverage to turn Walters and Bloom into informants against their underworld associates.

ONE MOMENT CHANGES EVERYTHING

Ironically, another man who turned heads wherever he went had already turned State's witness. Despite serving concurrent nine-year prison sentences for racketeering and tax evasion, former Colombo Crime Family captain Michael Franzese was brought in to testify against Walters and Bloom under federal immunity. Franzese was the ultimate Mafia insider, but his past was hardly above reproach, and he wasn't exactly what anyone could call a "reliable witness." Already indicted numerous times, though never convicted, Franzese was the focus of a massive multi-agency task force, which had the sole purpose of bringing him to justice. Apparently, at the urging of his new wife, Franzese had turned himself over to Manhattan Federal Prosecutor Rudy Giuliani voluntarily.

The dapper Franzese invoked curiosity from outsiders, and a stark, sudden hush overwhelmed the court when he was called to the witness stand on March 15, 1989. Handsome, thick, athletic, tough—Franzese was known as the "Yuppie Don" for his expensive suits, and he cultivated the image of a mafia kingpin.

In his federal testimony against Norby Walters and Lloyd Bloom, the highly intelligent Franzese expertly controlled the court by not implicating anyone he didn't want to implicate. He admitted having had a long relationship with Walters. He admitted helping Walters remain the booking agent for Dionne Warwick (as well as Luther Vandross and Kool and the Gang) even after Warwick's manager sought to fire Walters. Asked how he did this, Franzese said that he simply spoke to the manager on Norby's behalf.

Franzese insisted that he, personally, had never applied pressure to any athletes to continue their relationship with the agents. Prosecutors then contended that, while Franzese may not have applied the pressure himself, Walters had no hesitation about using the Mafioso's name in threats on numerous occasions.

Walters' attorney cross-examined Franzese and challenged his credibility, but how successful that ploy would be was uncertain. Nonetheless, by willingly associating himself with Walters and Bloom, Franzese's testimony was damaging the defense's case.

THE ALL-AMERICA TRAGEDY OF DON ROGERS

Though he readily admitted lying to authorities in depositions given in 1986—when Franzese neglected to mention that he had holdings in Walters' agency—none of that seemed to matter.

"At the time," he clarified, "being a member of a organized-crime family did not allow me to tell the truth."

Franzese was articulate and believable, and besides, all he was saying was: the three were in business together. When the jury considered what that meant—that mob-backed agents were recruiting and dealing with college kids—chills surely ran up the spines of the Midwestern Americans filling the jury box. Yet, after a five-week trial and 40 hours of deliberation, the jury had reached a verdict.

Norby Walters and Lloyd Bloom were found guilty of five counts of racketeering and defrauding colleges based on payments and gifts given to college football players totaling approximately $800,000.

Several players called to testify had attended the University of Michigan or Purdue University. Interestingly, the University of Iowa, which the government had initially listed amongst the most seriously aggrieved institutions, ultimately was disassociated from the case. During the trial, the defense had revealed that federal witness and former Iowa star Devon Mitchell—the teammate who Reggie had been following that tragic night—had achieved such a poor academic record during college that he should not have been eligible to play in any games, and thus the university had not been defrauded. The announcement that the University of Iowa would not be entitled to restitution, federal prosecutors lent credence to the public's perception that charges against Walters and Bloom were founded on moral grounds.

The simple case was, Michigan and Purdue were awarded money because their implicated athletes had been students in good standing. Essentially, defense attorneys managed to convince the jury that Mitchell, as well as former Iowa teammate Ronnie Harmon—who, after fumbling four times and dropping an easy touchdown pass, in the 1986 Rose Bowl versus UCLA had been accused by some journalists of actually throwing the game—had been manipulated by Iowa in a similar fashion to how Walters and Bloom had exploited them.

Still, the jury's decisions regarding Mitchell and Harmon were the lone bright spots for the defense, which saw little else go its way. Upon hearing the guilty verdicts, Lloyd Bloom broke down and cried. Norby Walters, ever defiant, announced, "We lost the first round, but there is another round. We'll be vindicated." At the May sentencing hearing, both men would face 55 years in prison and hundreds of thousands of dollars in forfeitures and fines.

At the trial's conclusion, U.S. Attorney Anton Valukas proclaimed: "Some people think we prosecuted the case to create a new law (governing sports agents). But it was initiated because we felt two people were involved in criminal acts."

While that may have held water at the time, history would prove otherwise. Laws were soon created to govern sports agents and oversee both athletes and sports gambling.

The government had won its case—at least this round—but many in the media aggressively questioned the whether it all had been worthwhile. Authorities had failed to make an arrest in the Kathe Clements beating; nor were they able to prosecute Walters or Bloom for defrauding a private organization, the NCAA, out of its amateur athletes. The case not only set a ridiculous precedent, but millions of taxpayer dollars were wasted as well.

The government had seized the moral high ground early in the trial anyway. Testifying for the state were Midwestern icons Reverend Theodore Hesburg, former Notre Dame University president, and Bo Schembechler, athletic director and football coach at Michigan—men with unassailable reputations. Both witnesses asserted that, if the nation allowed agents to influence college athletics, gambling, blackmail, point-shaving, and organized crime would corrupt their purity while completely undermining the public's faith in college sports and the American way of life.

Of course, the jury disapproved of the agents' cynical view of America right from the start. Walters and Bloom seemed to believe that whatever they get away with was fair game—they'd even consulted lawyers before approaching any players to confirm that they would be breaking no existing laws by paying athletes. Yet, Michael Franzese's testimony and his mobster history were enough to enforce a karmic exactor for the agents' shady lives.

The jury chose to convict the men to send a message: Just because Walters and Bloom had found a legal loophole, no one would be granted a free pass to exploit naïve athletes out of their money or eligibility, or defraud universities of their financial aid.

On June 20, Walters and Bloom, surrounded by their defense teams, stood before United States District Court Judge George M. Marovich and pleaded for leniency. Bloom's attorney, Dan Webb, noted that National Football League commissioner, Pete Rozelle, who was once general manager of the Los Angeles Rams, had signed Louisiana State University star running back Billy Cannon to a secret contract before the player's college football career had ended. But the pleas and arguments fell on deaf ears.

Marovich sentenced Walters to five years in prison, followed by five years probation, while Bloom received three and three.

Afterward, Marovich issued the following statement:

> "If Mr. Walters and Mr. Bloom are guilty, so too may be many alumni, boosters, and coaches. I want to give fair warning to people who violate the rules. You may be playing in a different ballgame now, and it may be hardball. There's a new player on the field—the rule of law."

Marovich then said he chose to sentence the two agents to prison—rather than probation or community service—due to Michael Franzese's testimony that he had first financed, then allowed his name to be used to pressure the agency's clientele.

"Michael Franzese is a liar!" Walters would say. "I didn't need his money to start the business."

Though they were convicted of breaking the most liberal interpretations of existing laws, Walters and Bloom may have felt they were unfairly prosecuted. But if anything goes on one side of the fence, anything goes on the other side as well.

ONE MOMENT CHANGES EVERYTHING

"I never knowingly intended to break any law," Walters would declare.

Both agents said they immediately planned to file an appeal that would keep them from spending any more of their lives behind bars. Unfortunately, one move that Lloyd Bloom had made was spooking someone; and appeals, retrials, and new trials would offer too many opportunities for disclosure.

Somewhere within that land of moral ambiguity where Walters and Bloom both seemed to reside, someone had begun planning Bloom's assassination.

24

As Reggie prepared for trial, because of Jackie's disappearance and Don's death, he was more associated with drugs than any non-addict or non-dealer in history. Alcohol was also a star, however. Reggie had a .14 blood-alcohol level—not falling-down drunk, but intoxicated. Worse yet, he wouldn't find a safe haven in Sacramento, which happened to be the home of Mothers Against Drunk Driving founder Cathy Lightner.

Confusion surrounded Reggie's rookie-year, one-month stay at that Detroit counseling center, too. Some reports may have attributed the hiatus to a nervous breakdown, but others were saying it was alcohol related. Although most likely the result of both, the rehab stint tainted Reggie, who not only had the familial history of substance abuse, but now the stench of instability as well.

For Reggie's attorney, Elbert Hatchett, and Oakland County prosecutor, Richard Thompson, the months leading up to the trial became a literal tug-of-war for public perception and political gain. For Civil Rights leaders, politicians, editorial pages, special-interest groups, and non-profit organizations such as M.A.D.D., Reggie's trial raised complicated issues of race, celebrity, and circumstance. Further muddling clarity and fairness was the fact that Oakland County is the suburbs of Detroit, not the inner city. That meant prosecutors answered to a demographic that mostly had the same skin color as the three dead teens, not Reggie.

To assess the avalanche of prejudice over drugs and drug users that existed in 1989 America, as well as the double standard separating wealthy whites and wealthy blacks, is nearly impossible today. A rich, black athlete and a wealthy, white C.E.O. came from two completely different planets as far as mainstream America was concerned. Few people protested a C.E.O.'s salary.

Is this due to sports' visibility? Due to most athletes' skin color? Because intellectual prowess is not a prerequisite of athletic prowess?

Or is it all of the above?

Reggie was the perfect springboard for political gain. By denouncing him, one merely targeted the crack cocaine of human beings. Reggie was the intimidating black giant.

Women hated the fact that he had crashed with a female who was not his fiancée.

Football fans hated the fact that he was a millionaire bust.

Racists hated the fact that he *was* that black millionaire.

Anti-drug crusaders hated the fact that cocaine was sprinkled all over his past.

M.A.D.D. and its supporters hated the fact that he'd drunk and then driven and then killed three teenagers, who the media described as "children."

The frenzy was vicious, oppressive. Soon a local newspaper anointed Reggie one of the top 10 villains in Detroit history—a distinction Reggie still holds to this day.

As for Kenneth Willett, Dale Ess, and Kelly Ess—the three deceased teens—they were hardly perfect citizens, not that they needed to be. Though one had dropped out of high school, all three held part-time jobs and were undeniably young adults with their entire lives ahead of them. People would rather believe that a child has the opportunity to live and learn than die from mistakes. Renowned grief psychotherapist Dr. William Worden suggests that, even though certain mechanisms help us cope with death, "Bereaved parents never fully recover from the loss of a child." Loretha Rogers could attest to that.

The tragedy belonged to the Willett and Ess families. Robert Willett, whose son was driving the van, demanded a public apology from Reggie, who was swearing that he'd already given one. Reggie claimed he called both families from the hospital, but

Willett denied that assertion. The media began debating what constituted adequate contrition, which wasn't endearing Reggie to the general public, i.e., the potential juror pool.

Everyone wanted a sense of understanding and, most of all, closure. Award-winning author and journalist Mitch Albom of the *Detroit Free Press* wrote an article attempting to summate how Rogers reached such a low point.

> "What sense can be made of all this? For months, perhaps years to come, people will say the name Reggie Rogers with disdain. They will assume he was a careless, hard-partying athlete, a bad guy who was destined to take somebody down someday. Perhaps. But he is also a product of a system that coddles the star and winks at his off-field shortcomings. Call him a classic example of the American sports hero—an overgrown adolescent who figured he had lots of childhood left."

Though Albom's words are eloquent and accurate, they still form a perfect non-resolution. Our society demands concise understanding, wringing its hands to express grief and outrage each time an athlete or movie star breaks the law. Celebrity downfalls make our mouths water, and we crave them.

Was Reggie a bad guy? Was he a good guy? Did he drive drunk due to depression? In the end, there simply was no answer to assuage our collective desire to know. Albom dissected Reggie's childhood and learned that he was something of a "friendly bully," who other kids couldn't say "no" to but wouldn't intentionally hurt a fly. Yet, Reggie was everything, good and bad, that most of Albom's readers would never be—a talented, troubled enigma.

In the end, the opinion pieces didn't matter. Those who knew Reggie truly seemed to like him. While driving drunk was inexcusable, millions have driven drunk and escaped unscathed. They weren't any less wrong, just lucky. His history and his trial made Reggie a difficult person to defend, but he might best exemplify the fact that we all hang from the puppet strings of circumstance and perception—and we are only defined and remembered for little other than our most recent actions.

Awaiting trial was not easy for the 25-year-old pariah. He was responsible for killing three teenagers. The standard was simple and just: If you broke the law by drinking and driving, you forfeited your ability to negotiate, especially if someone was hurt or, God forbid, died—even if those hurt or killed were drinking as well.

When Reggie's twins were born, he could hold one in either of his giant palms. Less than a year old now, they were getting him through each day, keeping him going. What a paradox: He had killed three kids at nearly the same time he'd become a father. Society couldn't let Reggie off the hook for killing those three, but should it exact punishment at the expense of his children by depriving them of a father? How long should justice take him away? Would there ever be enough time to reconcile the pain he'd caused those two families?

Reggie threw himself into parenting, trying his best to become the kind of father he knew every child needed: One diaper at a time, one feeding at a time, one bottle at a time. That's how he got through each day—forgetting his destroyed career, the brother he lost three years earlier, and the deaths of three strangers on that dark parkway by focusing on Regina and Reggie Jr. A human being's will to live is astoundingly powerful. Few could survive what Reggie was going through, despite his responsibility or what people thought; and it was far from done.

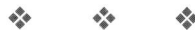

Media swarmed the trial, as 100 credentials were requested; but notoriety, skepticism, and analysis only meant that finding a fair and impartial jury would be difficult for Reggie. Elbert Hatchett requested a change of venue on his client's behalf because public opinion polls indicated that a strong majority of Detroit-area residents believed that Reggie should hang. Nonetheless, the change of venue motion was summarily denied.

Rarely would Detroit-area prosecutors have a case so rife with opportunity for recognition and advancement—throwing the book at Reggie could only help their careers.

Yet, none of this made Reggie any less guilty, or any more innocent. For some, Reggie was a potential pawn in their own games. For others, Reggie was the ultimate stepping-stone, the chance of a lifetime. For Reggie, the trial was nothing short of the biggest fight of his life.

To keep the three deceased teenagers from being put on trial, authorities refused to release their blood-alcohol levels. Besides being underaged, however, already information had leaked that the three were intoxicated, that marijuana was found at the scene, and that the street had been littered with beer cans—both having originated from the van. None of that seemed to matter to Oakland County prosecutor Richard Thompson, though. Two different judges assigned to the case had repeatedly rebuffed Thompson's insistence that Reggie be charged with three counts of involuntary manslaughter—a possible 45-year sentence. Precedence and circumstance both pointed to three counts of negligent homicide as the most applicable charges, especially with the State's burden of proof.

Some called Richard Thompson a crusader; others called him a zealot. Known as a hard-line conservative who hated plea bargaining, he would soon gain international fame for prosecuting suicide doctor Jack Kevorkian, who called Thompson a Nazi. (Kevorkian would not be released from prison until June 2007). In 1996, Thompson would be voted out of office for that same zeal, as taxpayers felt he used too much money pursuing ideological convictions. In 1999, he would found the Thomas More Law Center, a non-profit conservative Christian legal lobby located in Ann Arbor, Michigan. As TMLC's acting president and chief counsel, Thompson pushed for school districts nationwide to adopt intelligent design to their curriculums, and sued Planned Parenthood as well. Back in 1989, though, Thompson had his eyes set on a higher office in the future, and he seemed to view Reggie Rogers as a priceless rung on the ladder to greater things.

ONE MOMENT CHANGES EVERYTHING

The trial's outcome was heavily dependent on expert testimony from the police as well as forensic investigators who conducted tests on the fateful intersection. The unfortunate reality, however, was that investigators didn't want to exonerate anyone—they wanted to assign blame. Their goal was to find evidence to convict, and Reggie was the only one left standing. While a public majority sought that conviction, a firm minority believed Reggie was being railroaded due to his race. A smaller faction, definitely not consisting of the Willett or Ess families, even believed that, because two drnk drivers had somehow found one another, perfect justice had already been served.

In September 1989, District Court Judge Christopher C. Brown insisted that he would no longer hear prosecutorial arguments for involuntary manslaughter charges, and assigned Reggie to Oakland County Circuit Court, where he'd stand trial on three counts of negligent homicide. In a single moment, his worst-case scenario became far less daunting.

The trial began in early November. Elbert Hatchett, Reggie's well-known attorney, would treat this case like all his previous trials, instilling his own brand of tension, levity, and dramatic soliloquy. A Civil Rights leader since the '60s, Hatchett was active in politics; and as a former boxing promoter, he was known as a courtroom pugilist who could punch holes in the prosecution's case.

From the get-go, Hatchett seemed to have the jury on the ropes, their knees buckling under the pressure of his expert litigation. Some were moved to tears when hearing all that Reggie had lost—his brother, his health, his career. Newspapers filled their front pages with Hatchett's hyper-articulate quotations. If oratorical skill and legal savvy alone could determine the trial's outcome, Reggie might have walked away with the keys to Oakland County.

None of that mattered, though. On December 9, 1989, after one day of deliberating, the jury found Reggie Rogers guilty of three reduced counts of negligent homicide, asserting that Reggie was only 75 percent responsible for the accident.

Following the trial, but before his January sentencing, Reggie returned to Seattle to spend time with his wife and children. He decided not to appeal. He just wanted it all to end. On some level, he must have felt relieved to escape the involuntary-manslaughter charges. Now, a slim chance existed that he'd only receive probation.

Around the same time, a *Los Angeles Times* article appeared, questioning the role universities played in exploiting athletes. Graduation rates for college athletes were profiled, and many were stunned to learn that several major athletic and academic powers saw their sports stars graduate less than 50 percent of the time. Reggie was interviewed for the article; but, perhaps a bit surprisingly, he lauded the University of Washington's support system. He believed that Washington had taken care of his needs by providing him with tutors.

"If they didn't make me [study], I would have gone right home and gone to bed," he stated.

Reggie re-enrolled at Washington for the winter quarter so he could complete his degree in psychology. He only needed 33 credit hours to finish.

On January 16, 1990, however—just five days before Reggie's 26th birthday, Oakland County Circuit Judge Gene Schnelz handed down three 16- to 24-month stays in prison—one for each guilty verdict, and the maximum penalty allowed by law—to be served concurrently.

As Michigan offender No. 206525, Reggie entered Brighton prison camp, today a women's facility, in February 1990 for a minimum 16-month incarceration. His body had healed, but inside Reggie had to be hurting. Not only had he lost his brother, his health, and his career, he had lost his family and his freedom now as well.

One has to wonder what Reggie thought about that first night. Did he contemplate his unparalleled natural talent? Did he remember tinkering in the garage, riding his bike over makeshift jumps, and building forts as a kid? Did he regret ever playing sports? Did he wonder if there was any other way that he could've left The Heights? Did he imagine his family and how he used to speak of wanting many children of his own to love and to raise with a simple life?

Perhaps he just thought of his twins, and how they were the only stars in the endless darkness that threatened to envelope him.

Prison life was routine and boring, but even mid-level security facilities can be extremely dangerous. Reggie wasn't an easy target, but prison was full of young gunslingers anxious to make a name for themselves and older, hardened criminals who knew all the angles. As a celebrity, Reggie undoubtedly had to watch his back at all times.

Early on, Reggie White, who had been drafted the same year as Don, came to visit Rogers. Because he had played in many of the college all-star games and was a member of many of the same All-America teams, White knew Reggie's brother well. Under different circumstances, Reggie Rogers was supposed to become Reggie White: a dominant rushing defensive end of unmatched skill. In fact, Reggie Rogers was a better athlete and faster than White.

Yet, Reggie White embodied everything that was good about the NFL. In an incomparable era of drug abuse, White was a pious family man, who, though often criticized for his ultra-conservative views, would never flunk a drug test or drink, let alone drink and drive. That he came to console his former comrade, that he came to help Reggie pray for the Willett and Ess families, says volumes about Reggie White and his legacy.

White breathed some air into Reggie Rogers' deflated shell. Rogers began making friends with inmates of all colors and creeds. He befriended Muslims, mostly because they don't eat pork, and that meant Reggie could eat their servings on "pork Wednesday." Making the most of his time behind bars, Reggie enjoyed a sort of "intellectual awakening" during his incarceration. He began to read constantly, devouring any book he could find.

Downtime had never been kind to Reggie Rogers, but faced with either self-destruction or creativity, he chose the latter. Taking advantage of the art supplies available to inmates, Reggie began creating picture books for his children.

25

On February 6, 1991, after serving just shy of 13 months in prison, Reggie Rogers was released to his family. The broken neck that probably should've killed him had healed, but he told journalists that he had resigned never to play football again. "My priorities are God and family," Reggie would tell a reporter.

Yet, just 20 days after being released from prison, Reggie signed a contract to play for the AFC champion Buffalo Bills, a team fresh off a 20-19 loss to the New York Giants in Super Bowl XXV. A few months later, Reggie was back at an NFL training camp that would foster the next three AFC champions. The Bills saw a highly motivated Reggie as the perfect counterpart to All-World defensive end Bruce Smith.

"He (Reggie) has a bright, level-headed wife who's been good for him," Bills head coach, Marv Levy, told *The New York Times*, "and he's become a born-again Christian. We hope it will work out for us, and we certainly hope it will work out for him."

An unconfirmed rumor arose that Buffalo Bills owner Ralph Wilson, a longtime Michigan resident who had lived in and around Detroit for more than 30 years, orchestrated Reggie's arrival in Buffalo. Supposedly, Wilson had shared a "society conversation" at a Detroit-area function that revealed Reggie had been prosecuted overzealously due to his celebrity and, possibly, his race. Supposedly, Wilson, a staunch Civil Rights advocate but not usually a meddler in day-to-day franchise operations, then went over his coaches' heads and went after Reggie the next day.

ONE MOMENT CHANGES EVERYTHING

Right away, several reactions popped up regarding Reggie's second chance. Reporters launched an offensive on the Willett and Ess families, who told them that Reggie had not yet exhibited adequate contrition for his role in three deaths, so they were suing him. When Reggie was asked to comment on the still-pending civil suit, he told *The New York Times*, "No one is supposed to die like that. But what am I supposed to do, become homeless, lose my family, become a junkie before they can see the remorse?" But everyone who had known Reggie or who covered professional football could see that the man had changed. Gone was the persecuted, paranoid young player, replaced by an unguarded, grateful young man who was amazed that he was even alive. One has to wonder, after all the tragedy that had beset him and his family, whether prison was just the thing Reggie Rogers needed the most. Unfortunately, three people had to die for Reggie to find his way.

After a Bills preseason practice, his body, still and sore from the rigors of contact after so long away from the game, Reggie slowly flexed an elbow as he confessed to a *New York Times* reporter, "This is the first time I can remember, since college, coming to practice without a hangover." Once again, he assured reporters that he has not had a single drink in two years. As they always had, his drug tests would come back clean as well.

Bills coach Levy told the *Times*, "This is a very talented guy. He's worked hard during the off-season, moved here, and kept a low profile."

Reggie faced more hurdles, however, than the simple matter of moving forward. Protestors picketed the stadium before the first preseason game—not the kind of attention a squeaky-clean, AFC Champion franchise wanted to cultivate. Signs denounced Reggie as a murderer and a criminal. The country's changing mores, however, had created fans who would forgive a player so long as he performed well on the field. Whenever Reggie made a tackle during the game, the crowd gave him a nice ovation; and some even stood and chanted his name after he recorded his first sack in over three years.

THE ALL-AMERICA TRAGEDY OF DON ROGERS

Trimmed down to a lean 280 pounds, Reggie once again was amazing coaches and teammates, who shook their heads at his combination of speed and quickness. He was a marvel—if talent were the lone factor in his success, Reggie could've been fine. That low profile meant everything now, and he had to steer clear of any trouble, no matter how minor. When Bruce Smith went down with a preseason knee injury, Reggie seemed a lock to make the team. He vowed to wear a black stripe on his uniform as a tribute to the three dead teens, but after a few preseason games, the League offices intervened and insisted that he remove the commemoration.

Battling numerous injuries, including a back strain that sidelined him for several weeks, Reggie played in just four regular-season games for Buffalo, arguably the best team in the NFL—one widely regarded as the greatest team in modern history never to win a Super Bowl.

Some of Reggie's teammates, though, wanted nothing to do with him. The locker room was divided conspicuously between those who welcomed him and those who shunned him. Even though many fans would consider it sacrilege to mention Reggie in the same sentence as Bruce Smith or Cornelius Bennett, at one point people assumed he'd become exactly what they were, or even more.

Teams, however, have hierarchies, and sometimes competition means less that asserting one's ego. Many professional athletes thrive on attention, and many despise comparison—their game is a job, and misconceived weakness can cost a player millions.

Many longtime Bills didn't want Reggie taking someone's roster spot, even if it was only as a backup player. Many perhaps were confused over why the front office had supplemented one of the top league's defenses with a national distraction.

Reggie was no fool, though—he saw all the cold shoulders as honest sentiments. He understood that the Bills powerhouse had something good going, and he realized that several felt his reputation could disrupt their delicate chemistry.

ONE MOMENT CHANGES EVERYTHING

One player who made his distaste for Reggie obvious was outside linebacker Cornelius Bennett, an outspoken team leader and league ambassador. Bennett went out of his way to make certain the Bills' newest acquisition was marginalized and ignored, and never once did he take the time to acknowledge Reggie's existence.

For Reggie, although he's a big boy, having the team's veterans welcome him would make all the difference. He no longer had Don, no longer had friends to help him alleviate the pressures he was facing. Now that team hierarchy accounted for everything, and while Bruce Smith and Cornelius Bennett were near the top, Reggie was undoubtedly at the base of the totem pole.

The talent-laden 1991 Bills obviously wanted Reggie to reach the breakout-star potential he had shown when the Lions drafted him in 1987. Too much time had elapsed, though. While being away from the game had kept his body young, Reggie's instincts and timing were off, perhaps permanently. Besides, protestors outside the stadium, as well as some teammates, didn't want him around at all.

After playing four games during the regular season, a day after Reggie recorded a sack; he was summoned to the general manager's office and told that he had been released. The Bills were a championship-caliber team who did not need to draw controversy. Reggie began to sink to the bottom of the barrel until Tampa Bay, a team that finished 3-13 in 1991, became desperate enough heading into the 1992 season to give Reggie another shot.

Led by innovative head coach Sam Wyche, the Bucs had a highly regarded, but notoriously ill-tempered coordinator named Floyd Peters running their defense. Peters was "old school," a very tough man in one of the toughest jobs in sports. Right from the start, attempting to extract the most out of the Bucs' new acquisition, the coach unmercifully rode Reggie. Former All-Pro defensive end Dexter Manley, arguably the most talented and infamous drug washout in NFL history wrote—in his 1992 biography, *Educating Dexter*—that Peters' confrontational style was part of the reason that he (Manley) relapsed into drugs in 1991 and was later banned from the NFL for life.

Perhaps, but if Reggie read Manley's bio, he'd empathize, while not necessarily agreeing. Having matured, Reggie understood that, at this stage in his career, being ignored was far worse than being criticized. "I'd get worried if he stopped cussing at me," he would say. Reggie had become responsible for his own life, and he knew that his choices had brought him to this point, so he chose to give Peters everything he had.

Some believed that, by signing Reggie, the Bucs had replaced one disappointment (Manley) with another. Reggie didn't use drugs, though; and he truly just wanted to latch on somewhere and earn a living off his talent while he still could. At 28 years old, that window was growing smaller with each passing day.

More so than any previous team, the Bucs were impressed with Reggie's work ethic and skill set. After spending the off-season working with the team's trainer in Tampa, Reggie had dropped to a svelte 272 pounds—his lowest weight since college—and he was being tested for alcohol thrice weekly. Coach Wyche raved about him to the media, telling reporters that Reggie was the Bucs' best player at training camp.

The team's best player? He looked that good.

When the familiar queries regarding his mistakes and family history started to arise, Reggie simply replied, "I try to put the past behind me, but I can't. But the thing is, I think I've become a better person."

It was a stark and uplifting message, and he really seemed to mean it.

"You gonna stay clean this time?" asked one reporter. "You gonna stay out of trouble?"

"I can't promise anything," answered Reggie, "except that I'm going to do my best."

Reggie was now aware that he couldn't change the opinions of others—that action spoke far louder than argument. To set that example, however, Reggie needed time. His answers to those tough questions did show one thing: He had realized that he wouldn't be able to talk or interview his way back to a better reputation. Perhaps Reggie was simply glad that he was around to answer the same old questions, even if he hated the fact that they'd never go away. Maybe he felt that he deserved to pay that penance.

When the coaches saw Reggie blow by a slow-to-react tackle on an outside speed rush, his actions sent a chill of hope up their spines. "Wow," they think. "Wow."

But, after all, this was Reggie Rogers; and his family's history, his own history, was all just too much to overcome with talent alone. The seemingly inevitable finally happened, killing the momentum he'd accumulated for his final run at NFL stardom. So close to breaking free once again, Reggie was pulled back down to earth.

Perhaps it would always be that way.

During an inner-squad scrimmage, a fight started between Keith McCants and Charles McRae. Scuffling, the two fall across the back of Reggie's legs, bending his toe up to his shin. He developed "turf toe," which any player would tell you is as debilitating as a broken foot. For the season's first four games, Reggie was on the injured-reserve list. Knowing that he wasn't a rookie with the world before him, Reggie rushed back, fearing that he'd be forgotten; but no sooner than he returned, he was hurt again. Tampa Bay had no "now" to consider—the entire Bucs organization needed to be reconstructed from the groundskeepers up, so there was no reason to hang onto a Reggie Rogers when they could use his spot to develop a rookie. Reggie was released upon season's end, and his once limitless NFL career had ended as well. Even though some teams were offering tryouts, Reggie walked away knowing that there were no more guarantees in life— or in football.

Regardless how one saw Reggie, he'd had a horrendous start to life; but none of his transgressions was intentional. He'd exhibited horribly poor judgment, but he didn't broker drug deals. He didn't stab anyone or help murderers flee the scene of their crime. Most importantly, he certainly didn't snort the coke that killed his brother. And while he had signed with three agents, he most likely did so because he was searching for someone to trust. The world had grown cold, and even giants needed safe havens.

It's a Catch-22. Had the gallant Don never been born, Reggie would have had to grow up earlier, and perhaps he might have been more prepared to handle the demands and expectations that came with his talent. Conversely, had Don survived, he wouldn't have allowed Reggie to sign with three agents, to become an alcoholic, or to squander entirely the many gifts bestowed upon him.

Hindsight couldn't change the fact that three teenagers were dead, though. Articles, books, rehab, prison, counseling, excuses, time—nothing could make a tragedy like that disappear for the victims' families. Yet, to define Reggie as a "monster" or a "murderer" was disingenuous; and to this day, he bears the Apollonian burden of his actions with shame. Yet, believing that Reggie was just a flawed human being like everyone else wouldn't comfort the Willett and Ess families—not one bit. Their pain was—and is—justified.

Forgiveness is simply too much to expect from people who have lost so much.

After returning home to Seattle, Reggie fell off the wagon almost immediately. He was soon charged with drunk driving and resisting arrest after a contentious traffic stop. The arrest rejuvenated his name in Seattle and Detroit newspapers. Yet, rather than further incarceration, Reggie was admitted to an outpatient treatment program after declaring that he was an alcoholic.

Reportedly, the Willet and Ess families were outraged, as was nearly everyone else.

❖ ❖ ❖

It's 1986.

A handsome young man—a professional athlete—prepares to take a shower as relatives fill the house that he has just purchased for his mother. It's a day before his wedding.

In this parallel universe where only good things happen, the young man pauses while undressing and thinks about the cocaine someone had given him a night earlier. Pulling a glass tube from his pants pocket, he rolls it in his fingers and examines the white powder. With a smirk, he tosses the bullet into the toilet, then turns the hot water on high and hops into the shower.

Later that evening, Don Rogers and his fiancée host their rehearsal dinner in Oakland, and then the following afternoon, they are married by her father before more than 500 guests.

The great day promises an even better life.

Later, they have children, and Don not only stars in the Super Bowl, but is elected to play alongside his younger brother, Reggie, in a Pro Bowl as well. The entire Rogers family and their closest friends from Strawberry Manor fly to Honolulu for the game. Don pays everyone's way.

One moment changes everything.

EPILOGUE

In early September 1990, the Illinois Seventh Circuit Federal Appellate Court overturned the April 1989 racketeering convictions of Norby Walters and Lloyd Bloom. The Court decided that the original judge had unfairly disallowed testimony from several people who had allegedly advised Walters that he was not committing a crime by paying eligible college athletes—supporting Walters' assertion that he had not intentionally done anything wrong. The Court also ruled that Lloyd Bloom should have been granted an individual trial, asserting that, if the agents were retried, they would have separate days in court. Though the decision would seem like a huge break for both men, all the accusations of backroom deals, threats and ultimatums, all the unsavory characters and payoffs, Lloyd Bloom's insistence that he deserved a separate trial surely marked him for death.

Chicago federal prosecutor Barry Elden, incensed at the reversal, immediately promised a retrial. Desperately searching for something that would stick, the government spent another year building a case. Many people were saying, "Why bother?" But the answer was simple: The government needed Walters and Bloom to get to their mob associates. The problem was, evidence connecting the agents to the most serious charges—attempted murder, assault, racketeering—could not be found. Determined to get a conviction, the Feds decline to pursue the aforementioned charges in lieu of mail fraud, which they were sure would stick.

During the ensuing trial, with Walters' attorneys expecting that conviction, he pled guilty to the charge of mail fraud in September

ONE MOMENT CHANGES EVERYTHING

1992. In exchange, Walters would serve 18 months in prison. Yet he was allowed to contest that guilty plea in the same Seventh Circuit Appeals Court immediately; and what was once a small victory for the government quickly became an overreaching case that was dead in the water. After all the accusations, the headlines, Michael Franzese's testimony, two trials, two appeals, and exorbitant amounts of taxpayer dollars, Walters became a free man in July 1993.

Less than two months later—on August 27, 1993—Lloyd Bloom was found dead in his Malibu mansion. He had been shot to death.

The case remains unsolved to this day.

In a September 1992 interview, Ralph Cindrich, a Pittsburgh-based sports agent, said in *The Los Angeles Times*, "It's no surprise at all—not when you consider the number of people he did wrong."

In his 36 years on Earth, Lloyd Bloom had done one thing consistently well: made people angry. His legal troubles as a sports agent were a mere fraction of his brushes with the law. Since the first racketeering trial in Chicago, Bloom had been arrested and sentenced to a year in prison for passing numerous bad checks, not paying his debts, and not paying his employees. The same underworld connections that had helped his sports agency thrive probably cost him his life. Yet, for a man like Bloom, outside his family few were sorry to see him go.

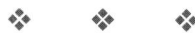

As for Norby Walters, whether he chose Hollywood or the city chose him is uncertain; but he continues to be successful at nearly everything he does while seeming to be almost everywhere at once.

Described as a music mogul, a super agent, a charity icon, an entrepreneur, and one of the greatest promoters in America, Walters has worked with Martin Scorsese, raising hundreds of thousands of dollars for the renowned director's Film Foundation, which helps to preserve classic movies. Norby's private poker parties, held in his

THE ALL-AMERICA TRAGEDY OF DON ROGERS

West Hollywood home, draw some of the biggest names in show business, including Sharon Stone, Dennis Hopper, Jack Black, Alec Baldwin, and dozens more. His "Night of 100 Stars" Oscar gala, a star-studded, must-attend, black-tie event that the *L.A. Daily News* has anointed "the number-one Oscar party" in Hollywood, marked its 17th consecutive year of existence in spring 2007. Walters' son, Gary Michael Walters, a graduate of both Princeton and Fordham, even executive-produced the award-winning film *Bobby* (2006), which profiled the assassination of U.S. Senator Robert F. Kennedy.

Norby can be seen in myriad photographs walking arm-in-arm with mega-celebrities, mugging with industry moguls, even standing beside politicians. Testimonials lauding his disparate charity interests and fundraising prowess appear in several newspapers devoted to Hollywood's happenings.

So how is it that NCAA headquarters in Indianapolis, Indiana, considers Norby Walters and Lloyd Bloom two of the most corrupting influences in college sports history? Norby Walters had cut his chops in the New York City entertainment scene with assistance from known Mafia associates. With their permission came the ability to run things his way, carte blanche. The fine line between morality and legality had become skewed—until Rudy Giuliani's vendetta as federal prosecutor in the 1980s, when he was able to weaken the mob's influence on New York's economy.

Simply, by navigating (and exploiting) those blurry gray areas that others feared, Norby Walters ascended from successful background player to legendary sports agent and broker. He saw the NCAA's hypocrisy concerning the corner-cutting universities employed to keep athletes academically eligible and used those peccadilloes to his own advantage. The NCAA, in the early 1980s, had attempted to institute a policy that it could not enforce. As others had done, Walters saw tampering with those still-eligible athletes to be good business because it wasn't illegal, as many others had done—he was just able to outwork and outspend the competition.

Norby Walters surely believes that he was a pioneer. Much, however, has changed.

ONE MOMENT CHANGES EVERYTHING

The Sports Agent Responsibility and Trust Act (SPARTA) and the Uniform Athletes Agent Act—adopted by 35 states as of 2007—has since been created. Agents now have to be certified, and they risk disbarment and criminal charges for defrauding the public if they approach student athletes with gifts or money. Today, the NCAA spends millions to preemptively thwart college sports' "dirty little secret," gambling. Former Mafioso and Norby Walters associate Michael Franzese still consults professional sports leagues and the NCAA, where he speaks to thousands of athletes each year about gambling's pitfalls and the dangers of putting oneself in a position to be blackmailed by crime organizations financed by illicit gambling revenues.

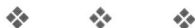

Former agent's runner Terry Bolar, somewhat more quietly than his former bosses, has achieved a high level of success as a sports agent, but not without peripheral scandal. As president and CEO of Prestige Sports International, Bolar has averaged two first-round NFL draft picks per year over the past decade. Mostly viewed as a straightforward, fair, and honest agent who represents his players loyally, Bolar today lists Bengals tackle and former first-rounder Willie Anderson and Bills running back Terrence McGee amongst his clientele.

Bolar was never charged in association to the government's racketeering and mail fraud cases against Walters and Bloom. More importantly, authorities never found evidence that Bolar had provided the cocaine that killed Don Rogers. Yet, amazingly, Don Rogers was not the only star athlete to drop dead in Bolar's proximity.

On May 30, 1998, Leon Bender, the 31st overall selection in that year's NFL draft, was found unconscious in the bathroom of Bolar's Marietta, Georgia home. Though rushed to the hospital, the 22-year-old Oakland Raider rookie was dead on arrival. Though the media rushed to assign blame to drugs, that proved not to be the case. Bender had battled epilepsy his entire life, and the

THE ALL-AMERICA TRAGEDY OF DON ROGERS

affliction was found to have caused his death. In response, Bolar immediately helped to establish the highly regarded Leon Bender Foundation, which raises funds to research epilepsy and attracts some of the biggest names in sports as fundraisers and spokespersons.

Today, Bolar's Prestige Sports International website still lists Reggie Rogers amongst his former clientele.

❖ ❖ ❖

Don the Prince has been gone for just over 20 years. Buried next to him is Loretha, who died of heart failure in 2000.

As an adult, the lovely, effervescent Jackie Rogers has continued to struggle. When reporters came around to pen articles on the 20th anniversary of Don's death, she told them that life has been up and down for her. Now an in-home care provider, Jackie has her "good days and bad."

Whether the Rogers' collective downfall, beginning with Don, was the result of genetic depression will never be known. Most sadistic, perhaps, is the fact that our collective understanding of the disease shifted shortly after Don's death. The question is, could everything have been avoided?

Jackie and Reggie readily confess that, although they have tried, they simply cannot exorcise the demons that were unearthed that fateful June morning.

Don wasn't trying to pull the wool over people's eyes to hide his flawed character. He was battling, not partying. He wasn't proclaiming himself "The baddest man on the planet," as Len Bias reportedly said the night before he died. Don was the first to leave his own bachelor party. He didn't run the streets but went home to his mother's and went to bed. Though he may have appeared "fine" on the outside—in control and able to handle the pressures of his seemingly "perfect" life—little doubt exists that he was engaged in an epic struggle against the expectations and hardships endured over his brief existence. Those who knew who Don was—Terry Donahue, Hanford Dixon, Frank Minnifield, the longtime residents

ONE MOMENT CHANGES EVERYTHING

of Del Paso Heights, and his brother and sister—know what he might have accomplished had he only lived.

Inside, Reggie and Jackie must sense what they themselves might have been were their brother still alive. They know all too well that one moment changes everything; and if that moment doesn't go your way, a full recovery may not always be possible.

"He was my bodyguard," said Jackie soon after her brother's death.

Over the past few years, Jackie has seemed hidden from view. At times, she's had an unlisted phone number; and at other points, she's had no phone at all. When seen around town, when reached for an interview, or—most poignantly—when she is seen crouching over her mother's and brother's graves, her presence is still that of a commanding woman. Her athletic talent and physical beauty not only captured the heart of Ernest Lee, the greatest high school basketball player in Sacramento history, but also a legion of devoted admirers.

"He is my bodyguard," said Jackie of her brother, Reggie, in a 2006 *Sacramento Bee* interview.

And what of Reggie? Giant. Controversial. Hated. To many people he's the classic, unrepentant villain—symbolic of everything that is wrong with sports. In the serious, working-class towns of Detroit and Cleveland, as well as parts of Seattle and Sacramento, he's the worst type of Benedict Arnold: a traitor to his talent, a superstar who threw it all away. All that is too simplistic, though. Reggie is a classic headline that broke free from the page, engrained itself in our collective consciousness, and ultimately became a four-star drama about the rise and fall of someone we think we know.

Perhaps the most vexing and flawed member of a briefly infallible family, Reggie today lives in Seattle in a world of his own design. His physical features remain handsome and youthful; his shoulders remain broad; and he carries his 280 pounds very well. But Reggie's demeanor is still serious, and the burdens he bore during his 20s seem to have carried over into the present. When comfortable, though, he can be effusive.

"He calls me now and then," says his high school basketball coach, Carl Youngstrom. "He talks, I listen."

He can be likeable, engaging, and polite—always offering guests the most comfortable chair and something cold to drink—but at the same time, he is wary and untrusting, traits no-doubt infused over years of uneven dealings with agents and reporters alike. Occasionally, when discussing his history, anger wells inside him, and his voice rises as stress mounts. Then Reggie will catch himself and quickly recoil, and it soon becomes obvious that he prefers not to talk about the past at all.

In many ways, Reggie's world remains remarkably consistent. He gives occasional talks to youth groups and goes to church. Ironically, while working as a phone-company electrician, he helped install the wiring for the Seattle Seahawks' new state-of-the-art football stadium, Qwest Field, proudly calling it "the best job he ever had."

Any peace Reggie has known has come from his family. He speaks with Jackie every day, but the unyielding restraints of his family history still shackle his ankles, prohibiting him from taking too big a step forward and, again and again, forcing him to his knees.

Over much of the past five years, Reggie has cared for his youngest daughter, who was born with lungs incapable of sustaining her life without medication, machine assistance, and constant supervision—much of which falls to her doting father. Her bedroom resembles an intensive-care unit, but she is obviously a fighter, surviving what few could endure. She doesn't fight alone, though. When Reggie holds her tight and rocks her, he speaks to her in a soft, low, reassuring voice. They coalesce into one being, and in those moments—no matter how many negative articles have been written or how many barbed questions have come—it is finally possible to see what's truly inside Reggie Rogers.

Yet, as if the battles of the present weren't enough, Reggie continues to fight lawsuits brought by the family of the driver he crashed into 19 years ago.

Maybe he deserves that part.

ONE MOMENT CHANGES EVERYTHING

❖ ❖ ❖

But will it ever end? The answer is probably "no," not when, of all things, a new generation of Rogers tantalizes the hope of positive headlines, scholarships, accolades, and stardom.

According to Glenn Nelson, editor of Hoopgurlz.com, the preeminent girls-only basketball recruiting and information source in America, in 2006 Washington boasted six of the top 60 high school players in the country. Only three states could claim more. Leading the way is Reggie's 17-year-old daughter, Regina, who was smaller than her father's hand after being prematurely born back in 1988. Today, she is a legitimate 6-foot-4 center and one of the most highly touted basketball players in America. Michael McLaughlin, who covers high school sports for the *Seattle Post-Intelligencer*, has called her "a spectacular talent."

Of 150,000 girls playing high school basketball in America today, Regina is rated as one of the top-40 players in the country. For the third year in a row (2007), her high school team, Chief Sealth of Seattle, was ranked No. 1 in Washington. Regina earned first-team All-State honors in 2007, won the Washington State Tournament Player of the Year Award in 2006, led her team to state titles in both 2005 and 2006 as well as a 2007 runner-up finish. Scout.com ranked Regina as the No. 6 center in the nation for the class of '07.

Regina has refined the myriad talents she inherited from both sides of her family tree (her mother Sheila's uncle, Chester Dorsey—Chet the Jet—is in the University of Washington Hall of Fame for basketball) to become a scoring, rebounding, and shot-blocking machine, who is all but unstoppable in the paint.

"I hope she's better than me," her aunt, Jackie, told the *Sacramento Bee*. "I hope she goes to Stanford."

Regina is the focus of an intense recruiting battle that surpasses the fights for her father, her aunt, or her two famous uncles. In an Internet era 30 years after Title IX was instituted to help create equal opportunities for female athletes to receive athletic scholarships—when women's college basketball has risen from

THE ALL-AMERICA TRAGEDY OF DON ROGERS

novelty to nightly television—speculation on where Regina would go to college was boundless. A "Regina Watch" sparked rumors about her pending decision that would last more than a year. Over 100 colleges were recruiting her directly, including Stanford, Florida, Ohio State, and Texas. Her family history, though, seemed to make the University of Washington the clear favorite, and Regina nearly committed to the Huskies her junior year.

Then Regina shocked Seattle and the college basketball world by committing to wear UCLA blue and gold instead, thus giving the Bruins a consensus top-ten recruiting class for 2007. Heading to the same university where her uncle was once Rose Bowl MVP, she will have the chance to join the ranks of John Wooden, Kareem Abdul-Jabbar, Troy Aikman, Ann Meyer, Bill Walton, and Don Rogers in UCLA's nonpareil hall of fame.

Yet, the disgruntled masses of pressure and notoriety have already assembled against Regina. In 2006, Chief Sealth High School had to forfeit its two state championships after the Washington Interscholastic Activities Association learned that Rogers was enticed to attend the school. The then-coach promised Regina and some other players starting spots and scholarships if they enrolled. Parents of opposing high school players prompted the Chief Sealth investigation, which one news outlet breathlessly called "the biggest high school recruiting scandal in American history."

Following her commitment to UCLA, Washington fired its longtime women's head basketball coach, June Daugherty, one day after the Huskies were eliminated in the first round of the 2007 NCAA Tournament. ESPN News, the *Seattle Times*, the *Seattle Post-Intelligencer*, and several other newspapers nationwide carried a report in which the Associate Press quoted UW athletic director Todd Turner as saying: "Quite a few kids have left our state to play elsewhere, which is troubling." Even though many of the state's best high school players committed to out-of-state-universities such as Tennessee and Oregon, the AP report named only one prominent Washington player who had elected to attend college elsewhere: Regina Rogers.

ONE MOMENT CHANGES EVERYTHING

In a cringe-inducing pattern reminiscent of her father's news conferences following Don's death, this 17-year-old girl now has her name strewn through the newspapers as part of two negative stories that will footnote her high school and college basketball careers: that Chief Sealth cheated to land her, and that her decision to attend UCLA resulted in the termination of a Washington head girls basketball coach.

When her family's tumultuous past is taken into account now and in the future, as her star ascends, Regina—as her father before her—may be forced to defend herself even though she has done nothing wrong.

What, then, has become of Regina's twin brother, Reggie Jr.?

When Reggie Jr. entered Chief Sealth as a ninth grader in 2003, he stood a thick and muscular 6-foot-3 and weighed over 200 pounds. As a basketball player, Reggie Jr. possessed strength, amazing dexterity, and a sensational nose for the ball. When basketball writers, scouts, and fans all considered his talented family history, they had every reason to believe that Reggie Jr. was destined for hardwood greatness. Then something unforeseen happened; or rather, something foreseen didn't happen. Far from a tragedy, but certainly a disappointment, Reggie Rogers Jr. stopped growing soon after his freshman year.

Most people would love to be 6-foot-3 with uncanny dexterity, but when your father is 6-foot-7 and your mother is 5-foot-8, you expect to grow taller than your sister. Not to mention, when your father and two uncles played professional sports, the pressures mount and the expectations are enormous.

The *Seattle Post-Intelligencer's* Michael McLaughlin has been watching Reggie Rogers Jr. for four years. Calling him "a truly great kid," McLaughlin cites interviews as well as examples of Rogers never argued a foul called against him and how much he enjoyed setting up teammates for easy buckets. He also says that Reggie Jr. is a fabulous player who has all the instincts for the college game and almost all the necessary tools—except one. As a 6-foot-3 post player, although a dominant presence who managed to lead once moribund Chief Sealth into the sectional playoffs in 2007, Reggie Jr. is simply not tall enough for the college game.

Nonetheless, he plans to attend college and be a force in life off the court. Medicine? Engineering? Law? According to Chief Sealth's athletic director, Michael Kelly, Reggie Jr. will decide soon enough. One thing, however, is certain: Regina Rogers has a fan club, and its president bears her surname and her smile.

One destined for future stardom, one destined for success in life, the twins—born just 18 years ago in a time of tragic uncertainty—are further signs that the Rogers clan is simply too talented and determined to blend into the crowd.

Once again, the family's momentum is building for a run at their American dream.

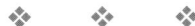

A little boy watches the door of the pizza parlor as he works on a slice, measuring one bite at a time. He wants to savor it, wants to make it last. Almost a year after his father's death, Little D still didn't understand what had happened. He'd been told, but what is "forever" to a five-year-old child? What is death?

Little D was certain his father would return; he always had before. So, on his fifth birthday, at a party inside a Sacramento pizza parlor, along with his grandmother, Little D sat and watched the door.

Later, Little D came to accept that his father was gone—too many missed birthdays to assume anything else. He learned to accept it all right; but the rest of Sacramento had trouble dealing. Whenever Don Jr. would go for a drive with Loretha, neighborhood natives would stop the car to tell Little D stories about his father: How he'd helped them out of a jam, how he'd inspired them, what he'd meant to the town.

"It crushed our world," said Del Paso Heights resident Connell Johnson in a recent interview with the *Sacramento Bee*. "It's still hard to understand and accept. Your whole life you try [to] find people as good as Don Rogers. We had him, and then we lost him—and you still find a lot of people around here who can't let it go."

Little D grew up knowing Don had been special, but did not know his father. That he'd touched so many lives, that he was a hero to his community was obvious. What he didn't know was how his father had died. That crucial piece of information came to him by accident; but in Little D's case, that revelation became the miracle that has shaped his life.

Barely a teenager, Little D opened his social studies textbook to find a full-page photograph of his father. He'd seen several pictures of his dad before, but the photo didn't accompany a list of great NFL safeties or UCLA All-Americans.

This page profiled the dangers of drugs.

"No one ever told me how he died," Little D told *The Cleveland Plain Dealer* in 2006.

Loretha had always told him that Don died of a heart attack, which was true in a sense. Right up to her last breath, she'd refused to accept that drugs caused her son's death.

Little D may not know it, but many people watched him grow up. In the 21 years since his father's death, thousands of articles detailing the tragedy and updating the principals have been written and rewritten. Little D was the only innocent victim in the saga of Sacramento's First Family. Many people—people otherwise uninterested in sports—scanned the articles about the Rogers for no other reason than to find out what was happening with Don's little son.

"Every time they run a story about the Rogers family, I scan down the page looking for information about Don Jr.," says longtime Sacramento resident and teacher, Dianne Battistessa. "I always have."

People are like that. They form attachments to the innocent. They honestly care. Yet, the best part is, if those people ever get a chance to meet Little D, they'll like what they see and hear. The soft-spoken young man is an anomaly in the modern world. He's intensely spiritual and hardworking but deflects attention from himself. Interviewing Don Jr. offers no glimpse that he was the focus of so much worry in the years since his father's death.

But Little D is as lucky as he is strong. While pregnant with him, his mother, Ajuanta, met and soon married housepainter and Del Paso Heights native, Tony Meadows—a young man and unsung hero who raised Little D lovingly, spiritually, and as his own flesh and blood. When asked how he could take on such responsibility so young, Meadows replied thoughtfully: "I just thought it was the right thing to do."

Today, Little D is 6-foot-3 and weighs over 300 pounds. Sure, he was a talented athlete; but finding that picture of his father in the textbook helped Little D find his calling; and he forever turned his back on sports. He speaks easily about how everyone expected him to either become a great athlete, like his father, or to use his father's death as an excuse to "wild out" and get into trouble. Little D just laughs because he followed neither path. The 25-year-old always had more important tasks at hand: helping around the kitchen, washing the dishes, taking out the trash, praying. At ten years old, he seemed completely grown. At 22, he bought his first house.

Today, Little D sings in the church choir. He's a highly regarded youth pastor who is working toward becoming a Pentecostal minister.

"I want to do whatever God requires of me," Rogers Jr. recently told *The Cleveland Plain Dealer*. "From my understanding, what I'm supposed to do is preach."

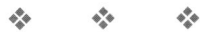

Perhaps somewhere in distant time and space exists that parallel universe for things that should've happened but didn't. If so, that universe matters because people like Don Rogers matter. Don was linked to so many worlds, and his decisions affected us all.

In the four years immediately following his death, the Cleveland Browns lost the AFC championship game to the Denver Broncos three times. Former Brown Hanford Dixon recalls the night of Don's bachelor party—when Don immediately pulled him aside at the Sacramento Airport and asked if he would ride along with him to the wedding.

Don said he had something important to discuss with his close friend and teammate. That conversation never happened.

"There's no doubt in my mind that, if Don Rogers was on our football team," former Brown Frank Minnifield told the *Plain Dealer* in 2006, "there would be a lot of [Browns] winning Super Bowl rings."

Many years ago, a brave young mother named Loretha took a bus from Arkansas of the Oppressed South and headed west to California. In her arms, she carried a golden child who would grow up to inspire the people who lived in his neighborhood: the toughest corner of Del Paso Heights. That young man went on to UCLA, where he led the Bruins to two Rose Bowl championships. Then, he went to Cleveland and led the Browns into the playoffs.

But then the young man died, leaving a devoted mother with a broken heart, leaving teammates and fans in Cleveland to dream of Super Bowls that would never be. Upon hearing the news that the young man had died, the Browns' tough-as-nails head coach, Marty Schottenheimer, broke down and wept.

The tragedy struck the heart of the nation as well—drug legislation, drug testing, drug war.

At Chapel of the Chimes cemetery, the headstone of a young man named Troy Scott Thomas sits a few short feet away from Don and Loretha's markers. Troy was a 15-year-old Del Paso Heights high school football player who collapsed and died of natural causes one year after Don died.

Embedded in Troy's gravestone is a glass-enclosed picture of the teenager posing in his football uniform. Young dreams of glory radiate from his clear eyes. Even 20 years after the burial, the picture seems unscathed despite all those chilly Sacramento winters and all those long, broiling summers.

Troy was laid to rest there to be close to his hero: Don Rogers. The two had met at a football camp where Rogers had volunteered; and from that moment on, the boy wanted to be a college football player.

Buried with Troy is his favorite souvenir: An autographed Cleveland Browns No. 20 football jersey that Don had given him at that football camp.

Troy Scott Thomas, like everyone else, knew how Don had died.

To Troy Scott Thomas, however, the "why" and the "how" were simply far less important than the "who."

INDEX

48 Hours on Crack Street 136

A
Abdul-Jabbar, Kareem 229
Aikman, Troy 229
Alarie, Mark 78
Albom, Mitch 207
Amaker, Tommy 78
Anderson, Willie 224
Anna Maria College 181
Anti-Drug Abuse Act 137, 139
Arizona State University 74
Arnold, Steve 118
Auburn University 170

B
Baldwin, Alec 223
Banks, Chip 91, 92
Battistessa, Dianne 232
Bedford, William 113, 181
Bender, Leon 224, 225
Bennett, Cornelius 167, 171, 215, 216
Bias, Jay 181
Bias, Len v, 2, 112, 113, 114, 115, 116, 127, 131, 132, 135, 136, 137, 139, 140, 157, 175, 181, 182, 188, 225
Bias, Lonise 181
Bilas, Jay 78
Buffalo Bills 213, 214, 215, 216, 224

Bird, Larry 113
Black, Jack 223
Blake, Marty 96
Bloom, Lloyd 163, 164, 165, 167, 175, 177, 178, 184, 187, 188, 199, 200, 201, 202, 203, 204, 221, 222, 223, 224
Bobby 223
Bolar, Terry 117, 118, 119, 120, 123, 163, 164, 165, 167, 178, 183, 188, 224, 225
Bono, Steve 54
Boston Celtics 113, 114, 131
Bosworth, Brian 93, 94
Boyce, Don 60
Braatz, Tom 171
Bradley, Tom 130
Brigham Young University 74, 106
Brooks, Rich 4
Brown, Christopher C. 210
Brown, Larry 42
Burney, Dale 8, 9, 17, 83
Butkus, Dick 76
Butkus, Mark 76
Byner, Earnest 104

C
Cal-Tech University 76, 77
Cannon, Billy 203
Carrier, Mark 58
Carter, Anthony 67, 68

ONE MOMENT CHANGES EVERYTHING

Carter, Cris 161, 173, 178, 188, 189
Cartwright, Bill 46
CBS News 136
Cephous, Frank 131
Chadwick, Jeff 195
Chandler, Chris 89
Chappelle, Ted 128, 144
Chicago Bears 76, 199
Chicago Bulls 56
Chicago Tribune 94, 136, 175, 176, 185
Chief Sealth 228, 229, 230, 231
Cincinnati Bengals 141, 224
Cindrich, Ralph 222
Clark (Atlanta) College 95, 96, 131
Clark, George Thomas 15, 19, 20
Clements, Kathe 176, 177, 178, 188, 202
Clements, Tom 176
Cleveland Browns v, vi, 3, 9, 80, 82, 91, 92, 103, 104, 107, 111, 117, 119, 120, 121, 122, 128, 130, 131, 144, 149, 152, 153, 154, 156, 157, 160, 172, 234
College and Pro Football Weekly 77
Colombo Crime Family 175, 178, 188, 200
Cordova High School (CA) 59
Crenshaw, Bill 182

D

Daugherty, June 229
Daughtery, Brad 113
Davis, Walter 181
Dawkins, Johnny 78
Del Paso Heights 1, 2, 3, 8, 13, 14, 33, 35, 38, 42, 60, 65, 75, 79, 81, 82, 83, 85, 111, 143, 162, 170, 182, 196, 226, 231, 233, 234
Denver Broncos 45, 157
Detroit Lions v, 170, 172, 183, 184, 185, 186, 189, 190, 195, 216
Detroit Free Press 185, 207

Dixon, Hanford 91, 104, 119, 126, 131, 158, 225, 233
Dodds, Tracy 48, 77
Donahue, Terry 21, 51, 52, 53, 55, 66, 68, 74, 105, 106, 130, 156, 225
Dorrell, Karl 54
Dorsey, Chester 228
Dorsey, Sheila 189, 191, 195, 197
Douglass, Maurice 199
Driesell, Lefty 182
Dubose, Doug 176
Duke University 46, 78, 88, 94, 150, 171

E

Easley, Kenny 21, 52, 53, 54, 55, 56, 57, 58, 59, 66, 69, 74, 77, 92, 104, 119, 131
Eatman, Irv 54
Educating Dexter 216
Edwards, Harry 151
Elden, Barry 221
Elway, John 157
Ess Family 197, 210, 212, 214, 219
Ess, Dale 193, 206
Ess, Kelly 193, 206

F

Fairbanks Elementary School 1, 4
Flagler, Terrence 177
Float, Jeff 15
Football Digest 92
Football News 77, 94
Fortier, Paul 63, 100
Fortune Magazine 175
Franzese, Michael 175, 176, 188, 200, 201, 203, 222, 224
Fryar, Irving 73
Fullwood, Brent 170, 177

G

Garcia, Aaron 5

Giuliani, Rudy 200, 223
Golic, Bob 131, 132, 155, 156
Gooden, Dwight 112, 181
Grambling State University 12
Grant (Union) High School 4, 5, 8, 12, 33, 35, 42, 59, 60, 61, 64, 65, 66, 69, 70, 71, 162, 178, 182, 196
Green Bay Packers 169, 170, 171
Green Bay Press Gazette 171
Green, Hugh 93

H

Harmon, Ronnie 201, 202
Harper, Ron 113
Harrison Narcotics Act 133
Harshman, Marv 47, 63, 78, 79, 80, 84, 85, 86, 95, 98, 99, 100, 101, 107
Hatchett, Elbert 195, 205, 208, 210
Heacock, Jim 108
Healy, G. Patrick 167, 168, 169, 177
Hesburg, Reverend Theodore 202
Hill, Aki 71, 79
Hoage, Terry 73
Holmes, Ron 105
Hopper, Dennis 223
Hornacek, Jeff 113
Houston, Gayland 75, 76, 77
Hunt, Tori 61, 70

J

Jackson, Jesse 113, 128, 129, 130, 131, 132
Jackson, Milt 4
James, Don 47, 80, 85, 87, 88, 90, 94, 108, 145, 169
Jesuit High School (CA) 15, 16, 24, 25, 26, 99
Johnson, Connell 231
Johnson, Kevin 45, 47, 96, 97, 98
Johnson, Earvin "Magic" 135
Jones, Rod 144

Jordan, Michael 46, 86, 113
Judge, Doug 101
Junkin, Mike 171

K

Karlis, Rich 157
Kelly, Michael 231
Kennedy High School (CA) 45, 46, 47
Kennedy, Robert F. 223
Kent State University 145
Kevin Johnson Foundation 98
Kevorkian, Jack 209
King County Department of Youth Services 108
Kornheiser, Tony 163
Kosar, Bernie 103
Krzyzewski, Mike 78, 150

L

L.A. Daily News 223
Langer, Michael 176
Largent, Steve 56
Lee, Ernest 45, 46, 47, 48, 63, 64, 78, 86, 95, 96, 97, 98, 99, 131, 226
Leon Bender Foundation 225
Levy, Marv 213, 214
Lightner, Cathy 205
Lloyd, Lewis 181
Long Beach State University 117
Los Angeles Lakers 114
Los Angeles Rams 4, 203
Los Gatos High School 40, 59
Lott, Ronnie 52, 53, 57, 58, 74, 92
Lott, Trent 138
Louisiana State University 203
Lude, Mike 141

M

Manley, Dexter 216, 217
Marino, Dan 104
United States District Court Judge George M. Marovich 203

ONE MOMENT CHANGES EVERYTHING

Marshall, Wilber 73
Mathias, Senator Charles 138
Matthews, Clay 91, 92
Massachusetts Institute of Technology (MIT) 76
McCants, Keith 218
McClain, Denny 112
McDonald, Tim 58
McGee, Terrence 41, 224
McLaughlin, Michael 228, 230
McMahon, Jim 169
McNeil, Freeman 54
McRae, Charles 218
Meadows, Ajuanta 233
Meadows, Tony 233
Mewborn, Gene 131
Meyer, Ann 229
Miami Dolphins 140
Miller, Cheryl 41
Miller, Chris 99, 100
Minnesota Vikings 184
Minnifield, Frank 225, 234
Mitchell, Devon 193, 201, 202
Modell, Art 153
Montana, Joe 54
Morris, Mercury 140
Morris, Ronald 177
Mosley, Roy 15
Mothers Against Drunk Driving (M.A.D.D.) 205, 206

N

Nelson, Glenn 228
Nelson, Kevin 83, 131
Nelson, Leslie 83, 104, 117, 127, 131
Neuheisel, Rick 54, 77
New York Giants 117, 213, 219
New York Jets 15
New York Mets 112, 181
New York Yankees vi
Newsome, Ozzie 91
Newsweek 136

Norte Del Rio High School (CA) 4, 5, 6, 8, 9, 10, 12, 14, 17, 19, 21, 24, 25, 26, 27, 28, 29, 30, 33, 35, 40, 42, 43, 47, 52, 59, 60, 61, 70, 79, 99, 122, 129
Northwestern University 92
Notre Dame University 131, 202

O

O'Brien, Ken 15
Oakland Raiders 224
Oklahoma University 93, 94
Oklahoma State University 106
Oregon State University 71, 79, 80, 107
Owens, Terrell 93

P

Palmer, Paul 171, 177, 187
Pascal, Blaine 168
Patterson, L. Brooks 195
Penn State University 140
Person, Chuck 113
Philadelphia Eagles 5, 51, 77, 188
Phoenix Suns 45
Playboy 73, 77
Pope, Dave 30
Prestige Sports International 224, 225
Price, Mark 113
Pritchett, Robert 95, 96, 131
Pro Football Weekly 77, 92
Professional Football Writers Association 92
Professional Sports Management, Inc. 169
Purdue University 54, 171, 201
Purnell, Oliver 182

R

Ramsey, Tom 54
Ransom, Cloyd 7
Reagan, Nancy 135

Reagan, Ronald 113
Rogers, Darryl 171, 172, 189, 190
Rogers, Don Jr. (Little D) 66, 73, 80, 82, 83, 104, 129, 131, 160, 162, 182, 183, 231, 232, 233
Rogers, Isaiah 162
Rogers, Jackie 3, 4, 6, 12, 13, 15, 18, 20, 21, 23, 33, 35, 36, 37, 38, 39, 40, 41, 42, 46, 48, 55, 59, 60, 61, 64, 65, 69, 70, 71, 73, 78, 79, 80, 84, 105, 107, 109, 111, 120, 122, 129, 131, 160, 162, 170, 183, 185, 194, 195, 196, 197, 205, 225, 226, 227, 228
Rogers, Joe 12, 13, 20, 83, 194
Rogers, Loretha 3, 4, 11, 12, 13, 15, 18, 30, 32, 36, 39, 42, 48, 65, 66, 73, 79, 81, 82, 109, 111, 118, 120, 127, 129, 143, 144, 160, 162, 170, 181, 182, 183, 184, 185, 194, 195, 196, 197, 206, 225, 231, 232, 234
Rogers, Reggie Jr. 208, 230, 231
Rogers, Regina 197, 208, 228, 229, 230, 231
Rio, Jack Del 73
Riverside Poly High School (CA) 41
Robertson, Marcus 57
Robinson, Jerry 77
Rockins, Chris 157
Rodman, Dennis 93, 113
Rozelle, Pete 141, 170, 203
Rozier, Mike 73
Rudin, Anne 130
Russell, Bill 96
Rutigliano, Sam 80, 91

S

Sacramento Bee 7, 15, 31, 38, 63, 70, 71, 162, 182, 183, 184, 196, 226, 228, 231
Sacramento High School (CA) 45
Sacramento Kings 81, 96, 129
Sacramento State University 80
Salley, John 113
San Francisco 49ers 51, 54, 56, 151, 191
Sanchez, Lupe 67
Sanders, Deion 169
Schembechler, Bo 202
Schnelz, Gene 211
Schottenheimer, Martin 91, 130, 156, 234
Scorsese, Martin 222
Seattle Post-Intelligencer 144, 169, 228, 229, 230
Seattle Seahawks 55, 56, 57, 92, 189, 190
Sharpe, Luis 54
Shrempf, Detlef 47, 63, 78, 95, 100
Sims, Billy 195
Smith, Bruce 213, 215, 216
Smith, Dennis 92
Smith, Onterrio 5
Smith, Steve 68, 69
Southern Methodist University (SMU) 177
Smyth, Dennis 136
South Natomas 80
Spielman, Chris 161
Sports Agent Responsibility and Trust Act (SPARTA) 224
Sports Illustrated 154
Stallworth, Donte 5
Stanford University 25, 228, 229
Steinberg, Leigh 177
Stone, Sharon 223
Strawberry, Darryl 112
Strawberry Manor 1, 3, 6, 7, 12, 13, 20, 42, 65, 80, 220

T

Tampa Bay Buccaneers 105
Tarkanian, Jerry 47, 95
Tarpley, Roy 113, 181

Taylor, Lawrence 112
Temple University 171, 187
Testaverde, Vinny 169
The Cleveland Plain Dealer 127, 152, 232, 233, 234
The Los Angeles Times 11, 48, 66, 68, 77, 105, 107, 127, 134, 136, 182, 211, 222
The Ohio State University 31, 54, 79, 86, 94, 161, 167, 178, 188, 229
The New York Times 134, 175, 176, 177, 185, 194, 196, 213, 214
The Sacramento Union 31, 68, 182
The San Francisco Chronicle 127, 182
The Seattle Times 229
The Sporting News 77, 190
Thomas, Russ 172
Thomas, Spider 46
Thomas, Troy Scott 234, 235
Thompson, Richard 205, 209
Time Magazine 136, 140, 151
Tribble, Brian 136, 188
Trost, Lonn 177
Trudeau, Jack 76
Turner, Todd 229

U

Uniform Athletes Agent Act 224
University of Alabama 161, 167, 171
University of Arizona 74
University of California-Berkeley 45, 51, 77
University of California-Los Angeles (UCLA) v, 8, 9, 20, 21, 23, 27, 29, 31, 36, 41, 42, 46, 47, 48, 51, 52, 53, 54, 55, 56, 58, 59, 64, 66, 67, 68, 69, 71, 73, 74, 75, 76, 77, 81, 83, 86, 93, 94, 103, 104, 105, 117, 119, 130, 131, 143, 149, 154, 201, 229, 230, 232, 234

University Colorado 54, 69, 105, 106
University of Florida 73, 229
University of Georgia 73, 74
University of Hawaii 46
University of Illinois at Urbana-Champaign 74, 75, 76, 77, 80
University of Iowa 201, 202
University of Kentucky 199
University of Maryland v, 113, 181
University of Miami 94, 103
University of Michigan 59, 67, 68, 69, 76, 80, 86, 195, 201, 202, 209, 211
University of Nebraska 73, 74
University of Nevada-Las Vegas 47
University of North Carolina 46
University of Oregon 99, 100, 101
University of Southern California (USC) 31, 41, 52, 58, 73, 74, 77, 92, 93, 94, 106
University of Texas 229
University of Washington 45, 47, 48, 54, 63, 64, 69, 71, 74, 78, 80, 84, 86, 87, 88, 89, 92, 93, 94, 98, 99, 100, 101, 104, 105, 106, 108, 136, 141, 144, 145, 146, 148, 149, 150, 161, 163, 164, 167, 168, 169, 171, 183, 228, 229
University of Wisconsin 54, 58, 69
USA Today 136

V

Valukas, Anton 202
Vanity Fair 175
Ventura Buena High School (CA) 70, 71
Vermeil, Dick 51

W

Walker, Herschel 74
Walsh, Bill 51

Walters, Norby 163, 164, 165, 167, 175, 176, 177, 178, 184, 187, 188, 199, 200, 201, 202, 203, 204, 221, 222, 223, 224

Walters and Bloom Agency 163, 164, 165, 167, 175, 177, 178, 179, 184, 187, 188, 199, 200, 201, 202, 203, 204

Walters, Gary Michael 223

Walton, Bill 229

Warfield, Paul 121, 122, 130

Washburn, Chris 113, 181

Washington Post 113, 136, 163, 181

Washington, Dwayne "Pearl" 95, 113

Washington, James 74

Waters, Maxine 134

Webb, Dan 203

Welp, Christian 78, 84, 100, 169

White, Reggie 212

Wiggins, Mitchell 181

Wilbon, Michael 181

Wilhite, Gerald 45

Wilhite, Kevin 45

Willett Family 197, 207, 210, 212, 214, 219

Willett, Kenneth 193, 197, 206, 207

Willett, Robert 206

Williams, David 76, 77

Wilson, Ralph C. 213

Winters High School (CA) 27, 28, 29, 30, 31, 32, 45, 87

Wooden, John 98, 229

Woods, Tony 177

Woodson, Rod 171, 173, 177, 178

Worden, Dr. William 206

World Sports and Entertainment 175, 178

Worthy, James 114

Wyche, Sam 141, 216, 217

Y

Yale University 115

Young, Steve 54

Youngstrom, Carl 5, 8, 9, 11, 12, 13, 17, 19, 26, 36, 42, 60, 129, 227

Z

Zucker Sports Entertainment Group 176

Zucker, Steve 169, 170, 172, 176, 177